single at heart

The Power, Freedom, and Heart-Filling Joy of Single Life

Bella DePaulo, PhD

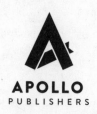

APOLLO
PUBLISHERS

Library of Congress Control Number: 2023930195

Print ISBN: 978-1-954641-28-0
Ebook ISBN: 978-1-954641-29-7

Printed in the United States of America.

To every person who is single at heart, this book is for you.

Contents

Introduction

Lovers of single life, set yourselves free! Unshackle yourselves from those old, regressive stories that claim that single life is sad and lonely. Rise above those repressive notions that everyone wants a romantic partner and if you think you don't, you'll get over it, and if you don't get over it, you need help. Gleefully reject the idea that putting a romantic partner at the center of your life is something you have to do, something that everyone wants, or that it is the normal, natural, and superior way to live.

I have a new story to tell you. It is based on experiences of people all around the world who are telling their stories, often for the first time. It is also grounded in social science studies of hundreds, thousands, and sometimes even hundreds of thousands of people.

My story is about people who are powerfully drawn to single life. I call them "single at heart," and I'm one of them. For us, single life is our best life. It is our most authentic, meaningful, and fulfilling life. It is a psychologically rich life. No other way of life will ever feel as profoundly satisfying. To us, living single is every bit as normal, natural, comfortable, and desirable as a committed romantic partnership is to people who are drawn to coupled life.

We are the curators of our lives. Being single doesn't limit our lives—it throws them wide open. We have our freedom, and we use it to make the most of our resources and opportunities, however vast or meager they may be. We get to decide the shape and contours of our lives, from our daily routines to life-altering transformations. We get to pursue our interests and passions, without trying to refashion or resize them in ways that suit a romantic partner. We get to welcome into our lives anyone we want—friends, relatives, mentors, colleagues, lovers, neighbors, spiritual figures, pets, or anyone else—as many or as few as we like, with no pressure to elevate a romantic partner above all others. We can devote ourselves to our inner circle, our larger communities, our countries, and our causes, if that's what we want to do. We create homes that are our sanctuaries. We have our sweet, sweet solitude. If we don't want kids, no partner is going to pout. If we do have kids, we get to raise them as we see fit. We enjoy intimacy on our own terms.

The risk to people who are single at heart is not what we will miss if we do not put a romantic partner at the center of our lives, but what we will miss if we do. I will never say that it is OK to be single, that it is better to be single than to be in a bad romantic relationship, or that it is better to be single than to wish you were. Those sentiments are far too grudging. For people like us, it is better to be single. Period. It is better to be single when we are young. It is better to be single when we are old. And it is better to be single during all the years in between.

People who are single at heart include women and men and people who identify as neither. We include parents and people who are not parents. We include the rich and the poor, the young and the old, the formally educated and the self-educated, people of all gender identities and orientations, races and ethnicities. Among our numbers are many kinds of believers as well as nonbelievers. Many of us hail from WEIRD (Western, educated, industrialized, rich, and democratic) societies, but substantial numbers do not.

The single at heart range from people who have never married, never lived with a romantic partner, and never had a serious romantic relationship to people who, in the past, have had all of those experiences, sometimes over and over again. We include people who are not at all interested in sex or romantic relationships and people who are quite fond of both. Some of us enjoy dating now and then. What we all share is that we do not put a romantic partner at the center of our lives, and we do not ever want to organize our lives around a romantic partner.

Perhaps even more importantly, we share the joy we experience by living single. Being single is something we savor. It doesn't matter if we have had no past romantic experiences or plenty of them. It doesn't matter if any such experiences were glorious, horrifying, boring, or a mixed bag. It doesn't matter if we had a miserable childhood or an exemplary one. We are not defined by any of those things. We are not single just because we are running away from something or because we have "issues" (everyone has issues). We are single because we love what single life offers and will continue to offer for as long as we commit to it and invest in it. For us, that's forever. We don't ever want to unsingle ourselves.

We realize we are bucking the relentlessly touted and celebrated cultural script that insists that what adults want, more than anything else, is a committed romantic partnership. We know what people think: that it's fine to be single for a while, but to stay single forever is just sad, and that to *want* to stay single isn't natural or normal.

Over the course of my lifetime, I've seen other bedrock beliefs pulverized. Is it abnormal to be attracted to people of your own gender? We know better now. Is a woman's place in the home? Oh, please. Is it only natural for women to want kids? That doesn't seem obvious anymore.

Each time our understanding of human nature becomes more expansive, we all become freer to live our best and most authentic lives. In the enlightened world that I envision, every child will understand, as a matter of course, that living single is a life path that can be just as joyful and fulfilling as any other—and for some people, the best path of all. Every adult will forsake forever the temptation to pity or patronize people who are single, and will instead appreciate the profound rewards of single life. Adults who are naturally drawn to single life will not be asked to defend that choice ever again. Millions of happy single people will realize that they are happy and thriving not in spite of being single, but because of it.

Because we who are single at heart are embracing our single lives rather than trying to escape them, we develop strengths, skills, resources, and attitudes that are less often honed by those who lead a conventionally coupled life. The time, money, and emotional resources that some other people devote to their pursuit of a romantic partner and then bestow upon that partner if they find such a person, we invest in the experiences that make our lives meaningful and that can never be taken away from us by a divorce or any other casualty of coupling. We value our friends, rather than looking past them for the romantic partner who may be on the horizon or waiting for us at home. Because we don't split the tasks of everyday life with a romantic partner, we learn how to cover everything ourselves, either by mastering each task, finding ways around it, or figuring out how to find people who will help or who we can hire. Because we plan to stay single, we create homes that will continue to accommodate, comfort, and inspire us as we age.

Our years of investing in our single lives and embracing all that single life has to offer payoff along the way, but the investment comes to its ultimate, stereotype-shattering pinnacle later in life. We've been warned that we are going to end up decrepit, despondent, despairing, and oh so alone when we are old, but that's not what happens. Studies show that it is the people who have stayed single who are most likely to be thriving in later life. Unlike the newly single, such as the divorced and widowed people who organized their lives around a spouse, the lifelong single people aren't trying to figure out for the first time how to do the things their spouse used to do for them. Lifelong single people never demote the people who matter to them once a spouse waltzes into their lives. They aren't trying to create a social circle or an emotional support system anew; they have been doing that all along. A study of older people in the United States showed that the men and women who stayed single were most optimistic about the future, were most likely to have an active social life, and most likely to have the help they needed and the intimacy they wanted. Black Americans, who are the targets of so much moralizing and shaming for their relatively low rates of marrying, were especially likely to be living a fulfilling life in their old age if they had never married.[1]

An Australian study of more than ten thousand women in their seventies found that the lifelong single women were not just doing better than the previously married women, they were also doing better than the currently married women.[2] Compared to the currently or previously married women, with or without children, the lifelong single women who had no children were the most optimistic, least stressed, most altruistic, and had the fewest diagnoses of major illnesses.

Those studies included all people who stayed single and did not distinguish between the reluctantly single and the single at heart. Once researchers start zeroing in on the single people who want to be single, the findings will be even more impressive. We already have hints of that. A ten-year study of more than seventeen thousand people without romantic partners found that, over time, the people who were not looking to unsingle themselves were becoming increasingly happy with their lives, while those who were pining for a partner were becoming increasingly dissatisfied.[3] Other research shows that single people who are not looking for a partner value their friends more, and as they continue to invest in their friends, they become even more delighted with their single lives.[4] Single people who yearn to be coupled often do not enjoy that heartening dynamic. The single people who want to stay single are also more sexually satisfied.[5]

I've been studying single people since December 17, 1992. That's the day I created a secret folder labeled only with the number 1 and slipped into it a clipping from an advice column in the local newspaper. I had underlined one sentence, "Remember that one is a whole number."

I was thirty-nine and single. I didn't think I was less than a whole person, but I did think it was curious that so many of the depictions of single people I would place in the folder, from Cathy cartoons to book reviews in the *New Yorker*, were based on the premise that to be single was to be sad and that no one would choose to be or stay single.

My obsession did not stay secret for long. Within a few years, I had mostly forsaken my previous area of expertise (in the psychology of lying and detecting lies), and completely immersed myself in my new study of single people and single life. Deception was an interest of mine. Singlehood became my passion. I conducted studies, taught courses, published research papers, wrote dozens of articles for newspapers and magazines, published hundreds of blog posts, gave a TEDx talk, started the Community of Single People Facebook group, and wrote books, beginning with *Singled Out: How Singles Are Stereotyped, Stigmatized, and Ignored, and Still Live Happily Ever After.*

I'm a social psychologist, a researcher and not a therapist, but over the years hundreds of people have sent me emails or handwritten notes telling me about their single lives. Two themes have stood out. The first one is dismaying. Over and over again, people have told me that until they encountered my work, they never realized that it was OK to like being single and to want to stay single. The second is more exuberant. Those people have described themselves as powerfully drawn to single life. They have effused about how meaningful and fulfilling it was to live single, and how nothing else compared. That's how I felt too. And that's when I realized that the popular narratives of single life just weren't capturing what it could mean to live single and to love that life truly and deeply. They did not speak to people like us, who were single at heart.

I was also intrigued by the single people who were pining for a romantic partner and the many pundits, essayists, and experts who extolled coupled life. Some seemed clear-minded, but many others seemed to be envisioning what I would come to think of as the Magical Mythical Romantic Partner. That's the person who is always kind, always attentive, always around when you need them, and always happy to do their share of the work. That's the partner who always wants the same kind and amount of sex that you do, at the same time that you do, and who never strays. As a parent, this partner is always present with your children and devoted to them, and the family you have together is free of conflict or cruelty. In later life, the Magical Mythical Romantic Partner is always there when you've fallen and can't get up. This person is there when you need a ride to a medical procedure or need someone to stay with you at the hospital, and is by your side no matter how long your illness lasts. This partner is never sick, and is never sick of you.

I don't doubt that some romantic partners, married or otherwise, truly are wonderful. But I also know they are human. As obvious as that sounds, I think it is a point that eludes the single at heart skeptics, who don't believe that anyone could want a life that is not built around a romantic partner. The partner they have in mind is fictional. For the single at heart, though, even a perfect partner would not lure us away from our single lives. We are drawn to single life by what it has to offer; we are not fleeing from coupledom because romantic partners are imperfect.

On Valentine's Day 2012, I posted a brief quiz online titled "Are you single at heart?" (It is at the end of Chapter 1 if you want to take a look.) By 2019, when I was ready to analyze the data for this book, nearly nine thousand people had taken the quiz. By 2022, that number had more than doubled to nineteen thousand, and it just keeps growing. The participants hailed from more than one hundred countries and every continent except Antarctica. Residents of the United States, Canada, England, and Australia flocked to the quiz. People from places such as Albania and Algeria, Egypt and El Salvador, Iran and India, Japan and Jordan, New Zealand and Norway, Russia and Rwanda, Ukraine and Uruguay—all found their way to the quiz and answered the questions.

The results of the quiz helped me understand, in broad strokes, how people who are single at heart differ from people who are not. But I also wanted to understand the single at heart more deeply. I wanted to hear the stories of their lives. I posted on my website, blogs, and social media a request for people who identified as single at heart to tell me, in great detail and in writing, all about their lives, and to allow me to quote them in this book. The forty-one people who agreed by the time I was ready to start writing this book include women and men, people of different sexual and gender identities and orientations, parents and people with no children, and people of different races and ethnicities. They range in age from twenty-somethings to seventy-somethings. Most are from the US, but others are from Austria, Australia, Canada, England, India, Mexico, and Portugal. (I'll mostly use first names only, either their actual names or the ones they requested. A few people have published books or articles about single life, and when I refer to those publications, I will use their last names too. The ages I report, as well as the places where they live and the other details of their lives, are from the year they described their experiences, 2019 or 2020. I describe their location however they wished—a specific city, a region, or country.)

My understanding of what it means to be single at heart has also been informed by the hundreds of people who shared stories of their lives with me more informally or told me about their role models, including people who are and are not single at heart, and by the results of many systematic studies of single people. When I noticed people expressing a single at heart sentiment in an essay, book, podcast, talk, or anywhere else, I added them to my files. They include everyone from the famous to the unknown, and you will meet some of them in this book too.

In early 2020 I thought I was ready to start writing this book. I gathered my copious materials and opened a new document on my computer. The date was March 10, 2020. The next day, Governor Gavin Newsom of California, where I am an academic affiliate at the University of California, Santa Barbara, announced that public health officials had determined that gatherings should be postponed or canceled across the state until at least the end of March. COVID-19 had come to California.

For the first time in all my years of studying single life, I had a crisis of confidence. The single at heart love solitude, but how would we deal with weeks of it? If there's anything we cherish more than solitude, it's our freedom. With a pandemic lockdown, spending time alone would not be something we freely chose, but something that was imposed. What if the lockdown went on for months? What if it lasted a year?

I stopped writing and watched as the pandemic threw everything it had at single people, particularly those who live alone: isolation, social distancing, masks, financial woes, terrifying health risks, canceled plans, work disruptions, and the inability to see friends and family. Would it send singles lunging into the arms of a romantic partner—any romantic partner—just for relief?

The ominous headlines began to pile up: "A pandemic is hard enough. For some, being single has made it harder," wrote the *New York Times*.[6] On Twitter, a sixteen-part thread was posted that began with, "I don't know who wants to hear this, but being single during this pandemic has been downright dreadful."[7] It went viral, and it was tweeted at me a few times. I got the message, and yes, I was worried.

Before the pandemic, the forty-one single at heart people who shared their life stories had been providing me with some of my most valuable anecdotal data for more than a year. Now I was afraid to check on them. Finally in December 2020, I began reaching out to them again, starting with the first seventeen people on my list. If all my high-minded optimism about people who love their single lives was going to get snuffed out by COVID, well, I needed to know.

I posed a slew of new questions to the people I contacted. The most important was: After nearly a year of pandemic life, do you still feel that single life is your best life? I held my breath and waited for them to answer. I did not have to wait long.

One by one they replied. Most responded almost immediately. Some had suffered setbacks, often financial ones. Many desperately missed seeing their friends in person and some craved human touch. Most were eager to get back to the "before times." But *not a single person* wanted to trade their single life for a life of conventional romantic coupledom.[8] In fact, some felt even *more* secure about being single than they had before the pandemic.[9]

They were thriving because they had already cultivated the kinds of interests and practices that turned out to be hugely helpful in surviving pandemic life. They enjoyed pursuits like reading, writing, meditating, and exercising, all of which could be savored solo. Many have long attended lovingly to their homes, and during the pandemic they continued to experience their homes as sanctuaries not prisons. The single at heart are used to taking the initiative to maintain their relationships with friends and relatives, and they are also accustomed to staying in touch virtually. Even when they were not seeing anyone in person, they were not socially isolated.

Many of the people who jumped on that Twitter thread about the dreadfulness of being single during the pandemic had one thing in common: they wanted to be coupled. For them, 2020 was a lost year in their quest to find a life partner. No one who is single at heart experienced the pandemic that way.

I was relieved to hear how the single at heart had fared during COVID isolations. I was also emboldened. Was it possible that some single people had gone into the pandemic wanting to find a romantic partner, but then changed their mind as the lockdown continued? I posed the question to the Community of Single People Facebook group. One person, then another, then several more described the lockdown as transformational.[10] During the pandemic, they told me, they faced their fears. They faced themselves. They found comfort in solitude, emotional closeness in relationships that were not romantic, wisdom in their self-reflection, and joy in both the new opportunities they pursued and the strength they'd never realized they had. Most significantly, they learned that single life was not just something they could handle, but something they relished.

The pandemic was a time of reckoning for couples as well as singles. Some couples have grown closer. Others have fallen apart. In "Covid Ended Our Marriage," the BBC reported, "All around the world—from South America to West Africa—previously happy couples are splitting up, and many are divorcing."[11]

The already fraught issue of the division of household chores became even more tense as those chores multiplied during lockdown. Many couples and families longed for what people who are single at heart access easily: freedom to do what they wanted to do when they wanted to do it, and time and space to themselves. The *Globe and Mail* reported on people sitting alone in their parked cars just to have a moment on their own.[12] In a work of photojournalism, the *Washington Post* published photos of "pandemic sheds" some families had built "to create room for silence, storage, and solace."[13]

New York Times reporters talked to people across the country about their pandemic experiences and in April 2021, they described their findings: "Over and over, people were reevaluating their most important relationships, where they want to live, and how they want to be in the world."[14]

My book project was back on. The single at heart had reaffirmed their commitment to single life by a once in a century natural experiment.

This Is Our Time

For more than half a century we have been in the midst of a worldwide transformation in how we live. Women have been having fewer babies.[15] More people are living alone.[16] Where nuclear families once were the norm, they are now less common. In at least twenty-five nations, if you knock on any door at random, you are more likely to be greeted by a person living alone than a couple and their children.[17] In those countries, there are more one-person households than nuclear family households. In some of them, such as Finland, Germany, Japan, and Estonia, there are about twice as many.

Central to the demographic revolution is a retreat from marriage. A United Nations report tracking changes between 1990 and 2010 showed that in every region of the world, a smaller percentage of adults were marrying, and of those who did marry, they were doing so at increasingly older ages.[18] Also, all around the world, a greater percentage of people were divorced in 2010 than several decades before.

The decline of marriage has continued beyond the years tracked by the UN report. For example, the Organization for Economic Co-operation and Development found that between 1970 and 2020, rates of marriage had declined for thirty-four of the thirty-seven nations for which data were available.[19] They included, for example, Costa Rica, Greece, Japan, Korea, Norway, Slovenia, and Switzerland. In every nation, women and men who married for the first time were on average older in 2020 than they were in 1990.

In the US, it is not just the rates of marriage, but also the rates of remarriage that are decreasing, a trend only partly explained by the decision of some couples to cohabit instead.[20] Although rates of divorce have slowed overall, they remain high, and they are continuing to increase among the over-fifty set.[21] All told, Americans spend more years of their adult lives not married than married.[22]

In theory, the decline of marriage could mean that the people who do marry are happier than they were when marriage felt more mandatory. But that's not what's happening. Every year since 1972 (when researchers started keeping track), couples in the US have been reporting lower and lower levels of happiness in their marriages.[23] That trend has not put a dent in the relentless promotion of marriage. In fact, the unabashed defense of marriage may have reached a remarkable nadir in 2022, when the Well+Being editor of the *Washington Post* proclaimed that "hating your romantic partner is 'normal.'" She offered tips on what to do about it, and the first was, "It's OK to hate your partner."[24]

The flip side of the decline of marriage is the rise of single people. In many nations, it has never been as possible to lead a full and fulfilling life as a single person as it is now, especially for women. Even though women often get paid less than men for the same work, many earn enough to support themselves as well as children, if they want kids. They don't need a spouse for that. Single motherhood still does not have the same social acceptance as married motherhood, but the number of single mothers—and fathers—keeps growing, and contrary to all the scare stories, most of their children are doing just fine.[25] Or more than fine. As I will show a little later, single-parent families have some rarely acknowledged advantages over married-parent families.

Want to stay single and still have sex? In many nations it has been a good long time since sex outside of marriage or committed romantic coupling has been stigmatized. If anything, we've teetered in the other direction, in which not having sex or not wanting sex is what needs to be justified or explained. Want sex but not children? Use birth control. Want children without having sex, a committed sexual partner, or a spouse? Advances in reproductive medicine have made that more possible too.

Want companionship you can count on? Want intimacy? No one needs marriage or a committed romantic partner for either of those things. Have you gotten married but now want out? Around the world, divorce is more likely to be legally available and less likely to be denounced than it was a half-century ago.

Not into cooking? You don't need a wife or husband or any kind of romantic partner for that. You can pick up takeout on the way home from work or just stop at a restaurant and have a nice meal with friends or with your own sweet self. Don't want to deal with those bothersome repairs? Check the Better Business Bureau listings for a handyperson in your area. Need medications when you are sick? In many places, they can be delivered. Are you older and worried that you might fall and not be able to get up? You don't need a spouse in the house for that either—you can get a medical alert device. It's more likely to be there when you need it.

I'm not saying that contemporary societies cater to single people. They most certainly do not. Most policies and practices are designed with couples and families in mind, and that needs to change. In the meantime, though, the possibilities for living single that are already in place should mean that more and more people are living outside of committed coupledom.

And in fact, they are. The UN report showed that in Australia and New Zealand, by 2010, one out of every seven women (14 percent) had been single (never married) all her life as she approached the age of fifty.[26] The rates were nearly as high for Latin America and the Caribbean (13 percent) and still in the double digits (11 percent) for Europe and North America. In the US, a 2014 Pew Research Center report predicted that by the time the young adults in the US reach the age of fifty, about one in four of them will have been single their whole life.[27]

In the US in 2021, nearly half (48 percent) of all adults eighteen and older were not married.[28] If single is defined much more stringently—not married, not living with a romantic partner, and not in a committed romantic relationship—then 31 percent qualify.[29] That segment of the population, the solo singles, has been growing too. From the way solo singles are relentlessly targeted with self-help books and other sources of advice on how to snag a spouse, and pelted with unsolicited offers from relatives and friends to "fix them up" with some other solo single person (as if they were broken), even after previous offers had been declined, you might think they are all desperately seeking coupledom. But in a survey of a national sample of US adults in 2019, the Pew Research Center found that half of the solo single people were not interested in a romantic relationship, or even a date.[30] The older singles were especially unlikely to want to unsingle themselves, but even in the youngest groups (eighteen to twenty-nine and thirty to forty-nine), close to 40 percent said they were uninterested in dating or romantic relationships.

In 2022 the Pew Research Center repeated the survey.[31] This time, they found that an even greater proportion of solo singles, 56 percent, were not interested in a romantic relationship or a date. If all those single people were saying they were uninterested in becoming coupled for negative reasons, such as thinking that no one would be interested in them, or even neutral ones, such as being too busy, then the rise of these solo single people might not provide any evidence for the rise of the single at heart. But when the single people were offered a list of possible reasons for staying single, they most often endorsed the most positive one: 72 percent said they weren't looking to unsingle themselves because they just liked being single.

No matter how many people in the US or any other nation in the world say that they like being single and they have no interest in unsingling themselves, the number who would flourish by staying single is likely much higher. The deck is stacked against people saying they want to be single and stay that way, or even realizing how fulfilling single life could be for them. We've seen this kind of dynamic before, when many people—including many women—came to believe that a woman's place is in the home and that no woman would really and truly want to be anywhere else.

Why We Don't Yet Know How Many People Would Flourish by Living Single

Imagine asking the women of Vassar College if they have any interest in careers or any other independent achievements or pursuits, or if they are only interested in marriage and children. The question would strike many of them as odd, even offensive. But in the 1950s, it wasn't unusual or insulting at all. A ten-year study of Vassar students (back then, they were all woman) concluded that they had little interest in achievement beyond being a wife and mother. In his 1962 book, *The American College*, psychologist Nevitt Sanford wrote, "Vassar girls, by and large, do not expect to achieve fame, make an enduring contribution ... or otherwise create ripples in the placid order of things."[32]

A few decades later, women were still being asked whether they agreed with statements such as, "It is much better for everyone involved if the man is the achiever outside the home and the woman takes care of the home and family," and, "A preschool child is likely to suffer if his or her mother works." In 1977, a representative sample of Americans (not just women, and not just the elite, mostly white, women of Vassar) was asked those questions and two-thirds of them agreed![33] By 2018, though, Americans completely reversed themselves: three-quarters rejected any notion that a woman's place was solely in the home or that women were hurting their children if they worked for pay outside of the home.[34]

All those years when Vassar women were saying they just wanted to be wives and mothers, and Americans were saying that a woman's place was in the home, many thought they were describing something essential and fundamental about what it meant to be a woman. Women, they thought, were naturally nurturant and suited to domestic life. Men were believed to be different by nature, more suited to life outside the home in realms such as work and politics. (The people who did not have the luxury of choosing not to work because they needed to work to survive, including many people racialized as black, already knew better.[35])

That essentialist view of women and men was belied by the social changes that swept through the nation and much of the world toward the end of the twentieth century. The idea that it is natural and normal for women and men to inhabit separate spheres now seems embarrassingly naive. Instead, it seems self-evident that it is natural and normal for many women to want to have work and interests outside of the home, and that men aren't fundamentally incapable of domesticity or uninterested in it.

However, one part of the old-fashioned formula has stuck. It is still considered natural and normal and superior for adults to be coupled.

Women are no longer expected to define themselves *solely* in terms of their romantic partnership status, but that status is still obligatory. Coupling is compulsory, for women and men and people who do not identify as either if you don't want to seem abnormal, unnatural, or inferior. Coupling is compulsory if you want to be accepted as fully adult, and if you want to be part of the Couples Club, where you will be respected, admired, celebrated, and privileged simply because you have a romantic partner. In places such as the US, marriage is compulsory if you want access to a whole panoply of benefits and protections; if you aren't legally married, you don't get them.[36]

When Betty Friedan published her landmark book, *The Feminine Mystique*, in 1963, she explained how limiting it was to have "only one model, one image, one vision, of a full and free human being: man."[37] Now, more than a half-century later, we are still deeply and unfairly constraining humanity to only one model, one image, one vision of a full adult: a coupled person.

I'm acutely aware of the reign of compulsory coupling in the US; I've lived here all my life, many of the participants in my studies of single life have been from the US, and many of the examples I will describe in this book are from the US. But the centrality of coupling to adult life is not just an American phenomenon. Scholars based in other nations or who have studied other countries have found the same thing. For example, Professor Sasha Roseneil of University College London and four other scholars conducted a wide-ranging investigation of how things were changing for groups such as women, sexual and gender minorities, and single people in four very different European nations: the UK, Norway, Portugal, and Bulgaria.[38] They examined laws and policies, social movements, cultural traditions, and the everyday life experiences of adults who were not leading conventionally coupled lives. They found that things were getting better for women and sexual and gender minorities. Discrimination against those groups was less often ensconced in the law. Everyday sexism and heterosexism had become less rampant. Single people, though, could claim far less progress. In all four nations, coupling is still experienced as compulsory. The couple norm—the belief that being coupled is "the normal, natural, and superior way of being an adult"—remains dominant.[39] In fact, some of the social changes that benefited other groups only served to strengthen the couple norm. The legalization of same-sex marriage, for example, gave sexual minorities access to legal benefits and protections they didn't have before. But that victory, and the doggedness with which advocates fought for it, further enshrined the significance of coupling. Staying single, for people of all sexual and gender orientations and identities, meant that you just weren't as worthy as coupled people.

Committed romantic coupling is no longer just something people are expected to do. It has been elevated to an achievement, a status symbol, and a ticket to privilege. It is propped up by laws and policies and social practices that give couples special treatment. It is burnished by media representations of coupled life as the good and desirable life, and of snagging a romantic partner as the one accomplishment that outshines all others. Committed romantic coupling is kept atop its pedestal by everyday interactions with friends, relatives, neighbors, and coworkers who cajole single people to couple, fawn all over those who do, and pity those who don't. Under these conditions, asking people if they want to be single and stay single is like asking Vassar women in the 1950s whether they wanted a career. Sure, a few will say yes and go on to succeed spectacularly, but for too many others, it will seem unimaginable.

Going along with the privileging of couples and the marginalizing of single people is today's "placid order of things." Many of those who bask in the glow of their own coupled status, and many single people who aspire to that esteemed status, would like the rest of us to kindly refrain from creating ripples.

I'm not aiming for ripples. I want to create a tsunami.

Rejecting Marriage Is Not the Point; Curating a Life of Our Own Is

The couple norm positions romantic coupling, particularly in the form of marriage, as the standard against which everything else is measured and found wanting. Coupling is what is expected of adults. It is what they are all assumed to want.

Let's transcend that way of thinking. Marriage does not have to be at the center of anyone's life. It doesn't even have to be considered. We no longer need to ask ourselves whether we want to marry or have children. Instead we can start with an open, expansive slate of what our lives might be. Then, within the limits of our resources and opportunities and privileges, we get to fill it in with whatever counts as most meaningful and fulfilling to us. If we want relationships in our lives, we can honor the biggest, broadest sense of the word "relationships," and seek connections—casual, intimate, or anything in between—with friends, relatives, neighbors, coworkers, mentors, or anyone else we value. We can have children in our lives—and not just as parents—or we can choose not to. We can fill our lives with deep reservoirs of solitude if that's what we find fulfilling. We can pursue careers or passions or callings, or just dabble in whatever interests us at the moment. We can transform the place where we live into a home. We can settle into our cities and towns, or we can try out different places at different times.

When we think about life as an open slate, people are not single at heart because they have rejected marriage. Instead, they have chosen single life. Joan, a seventy-three-year-old retired professor from Newark, Delaware, who is one of the many single at heart people who shared their life stories with me for this book, explained it this way:

> For me, being single isn't a matter of not wanting to be married, any more than I became a professor because I didn't want to be a surgeon, or a pilot. I did not in fact want to be either of those things, any more than I wanted a whole lot of other possible careers. I wanted to be a professor because I wanted to be a professor. And I'm happy being single because that's who I am.

From the Most Privileged to the Most Disadvantaged, We Are United in Our Commitment to Be True to Ourselves

In 1994 Jane Mattes published *Single Mothers by Choice: A Guidebook for Single Women Who Are Considering or Have Chosen Motherhood*. The designation caught on, and more and more women began identifying as single mothers by choice. Many of those women were white, straight, and financially secure. They have been criticized, fairly or not, as using the label to separate themselves from queer, poor, or younger women of color, who, by implication, are stuck with single motherhood rather than choosing it.

My goal is just the opposite. I want "single at heart" to be an inclusive category, and not just a privileged class of single people. And in fact, many people who are members of devalued or disadvantaged groups identify as single at heart. For example, people who are single at heart are more likely than those who are not single at heart to be members of sexual or gender minorities. The single at heart are more likely to be agnostic or atheists. They are no more likely to be white, wealthy, or employed, analyses of the quiz data showed.

When I compare the single at heart to people who are not single at heart, I am not comparing people who want to be single with people who are stuck with it. I'm comparing people with different values and aspirations. The single at heart want to be single. People who are not single at heart want to be coupled or they already are coupled. No one needs to make the case for people who are not single at heart. They want what they are supposed to want. Their desires and aspirations are considered normal, natural, and superior. I am claiming equal legitimacy for all those who feel, in a deep sense, that single is who they really are, that single life is *their* best life—not just for a while, but for good. Maybe they deserve even greater recognition because they are persisting in embracing their best life even though they are too often stereotyped, stigmatized, marginalized, and disadvantaged for doing so.

This Book Is for You

People don't usually write to advice columnists when everything in their life is exactly the way they want it to be, but "Happy Singleness" did just that when she sought counsel from the *Washington Post*'s Carolyn Hax. "I have meaningful work, a home I love, good relationships with my three grown children, and excellent friends," she shared.[40] The problem?

> My children are suggesting I should be dating. And suddenly I'm noticing so much societal pressure to pair off. Even articles/books/blogs about happy single life/traveling/social life all seem to say: do these things and then *you'll be ready when Mr. Right comes along.* But I am happy now. Dates are fine, but usually I come home thinking I would have been happier reading a book. Still I wonder: will I stay this happy? Would it be better to have a partner in my golden years? Should I put some effort into finding one?[41]

If it is not clear just how stunning that question is, do something I will advise you to do throughout this book—*flip the script* and imagine a married person asking something comparable: "I have been married for eight years. My life is really good. My marriage is really good. I have a home I love and good relationships with my kids. But I wonder: will I stay this happy? Would it be better to split up now so that I have enough time to invest in a life of my own? That way, I could nurture relationships with all the adults who matter to me rather than focusing primarily on just one person. I could develop the skills and strategies I will need to live my life fully and joyfully, no matter who is or is not around. Should I put more effort into living on my own?"

That sort of inquiry seems inconceivable. But it shouldn't be. I don't mean that I want to encourage divorce among those who are happily married; I don't. But I do want to revolutionize the way we think about being single.

"Happy Singleness" was right about the books, articles, and blogs that seem to be offering an upbeat view of single life, only to end up rather grudging about the matter. We should stay single, they tell us, while we ready ourselves for the time when our real lives begin (or begin again), when "the right person" comes along.

All those writers, steeped in the prevailing narratives of what it means to be single, are talking past the millions of people who want something different, something that describes and validates their experiences and makes them feel seen. This book is dedicated to all the people craving a more enlightened understanding of single life.

Single at Heart is for the millions of people like "Happy Singleness" who do not need instructions on how to be happily single because they already have been for years. People who are happier reading a book than going out on a date. People who have great friends, meaningful work, a home they love, and no interest in coupling. People who are even more certain than "Happy Singleness" that single life is their best life. This book is the validation and celebration they have deserved all along, but probably never got.

Single at Heart is for the young adults who feel pressure to date, who may even have dating apps on their phones, but who, deep down, don't want to. They tell themselves they are going to get to it, they tell others they are interested in finding someone, but really, they like their lives just the way they are. It is also for the young adults who really are using the apps to find dates, but who still feel a stronger pull toward single life.

Single at Heart is for the not-quite-as-young adults who are closing in on that time when finding a partner and starting a family is the next step, the step their parents are probably pressuring them to take, and that some of their friends have already taken. They aren't interested but wonder whether they can trust themselves to continue to feel that way. They might feel alone in their reluctance, but they shouldn't. In 2018, when Match asked single women, ages thirty to forty-five, to name the number one priority in their lives, getting married did not even make it into the top three.[42] Living on their own (44 percent), establishing a career (34 percent), and achieving financial security (27 percent) all mattered more.

Single at Heart is for the people who are attracted to single life, but who have kids or want kids, and wonder if living single could still be fulfilling with children in the picture. The scare stories they have heard about the supposed risks to children of being raised by an unmarried parent may weigh on them as well. Later, I will have a different story to tell.

Single at Heart is for the young, the old, and everyone in between who has tried marriage or romantic partnering only to be disappointed every time. They were promised happiness, meaning, and fulfillment that would surpass anything they had experienced or would experience in single life, but never found it. Maybe the problem is that they never gave single life a chance. If they did, maybe some would find true love—the love of single life. The kind of love that lasts.

Single at Heart is for people who tried conventional coupled life and loved it. Maybe they had a spouse and kids who they loved. Maybe they even loved their in-laws. But now the spouse is gone, the kids are grown, and they want a whole different life. A single life.

Single at Heart is for the people who are in romantic partnerships and want to stay in them, but who want to break free of the conventions of romantic life. Perhaps they want to value their relationships with their friends and relatives as much or even more than their romantic partnerships. Maybe they want much more independence and solitude than coupled people are expected to want. I think they will discover a real kinship with the single at heart. Some may even end up identifying that way themselves.

Single at Heart is for the people who never will fully identify as single at heart, but aspire to learn from the attitudes, values, and practices of people who love single life more than they ever will. Even people who don't want to stay single want their single years to be as meaningful and fulfilling as they can possibly be.

Single at Heart is for our allies, including people who are coupled and want to stay that way. They believe that people who want to be single should get to do so joyfully and unapologetically, with the same benefits, protections, and privileges as anyone who pursues coupledom gets. This book will offer guidance on how they can best support the single at heart.

Single at Heart is for the one-time romantic partners of the single at heart who could never figure out what went wrong. Maybe they loved their person and that person really did love them. They tried to be kind, gracious, and understanding, but the relationship still didn't last. Maybe their single at heart person said, "It's not you, it's me." They should know that an explanation like that is not a polite dodge, it's the truth. People who are single at heart are never going to feel like they are living their best life if they try to put a romantic partner at the center of it, and that really isn't their partner's fault.

Single at Heart is also for the parents of grown children who are single at heart. This one is personal.

As I write this, I am sixty-nine years old, living in Summerland, California, and I've been single my whole life. I live alone and don't have kids or pets. I had a few romantic relationships with men when I was very young. I would have been truer to myself if I'd had none at all. I wake up every day feeling immensely grateful that I get to live this single life that I cherish.

For the first forty-five years of my life, my mother never said a word about my single status. In the seven years she lived after my father died, we occasionally traveled together, just the two of us, and we spent some holidays together. We talked about a lot of things, but she never pressured me to marry, not even subtly. I was proud of that. I thought it meant that she could see that staying single wasn't an issue for me. I never complained about it, collected bridal magazines, or mused dreamily about some future prince. I had an engaging career. In Charlottesville, where I taught at the University of Virginia for several decades, I owned a home that I loved. I've always had close friends, and she met many of them.

In the last conversation I had alone with her, as she lay dying, she brought up my single life for the first time. "I worry about you," she said.

I don't remember what I said in response, but I do remember that I was stunned and saddened. I wish she had understood that for me, and the millions like me, staying single was how I stayed happy and fulfilled. I wish I knew then what I know now and could have helped her to understand. I wish I had already written this book.

1

Are You Single at Heart?

"How do you know if you were meant to be single?" It's a question I've been asked many times. Sometimes it comes from a place of anguish, from people who are powerfully drawn to single life, but worry that their preference means something is wrong with them. Other times the people posing the question sound relieved, as if they've realized for the first time that maybe there's nothing wrong with them at all. I want them to feel something even better than relief, because single life, for people who flourish when single, is a *joyful, psychologically rich,* and *authentic* life. I want them to feel proud.

I don't use the phrase "meant to be single," because it suggests a whiff of judgment, as if the people in question are stuck being single because they just don't have what it takes to be coupled. People I call "single at heart" are, like those "meant to be single," destined to be single, but for all the best reasons.

Mary, a thirty-three-year-old from Buffalo, New York, said, "I identify as single at heart because I live my best life when I'm single. By best life I mean that I am thriving, able to be the happiest, most genuine version of myself." For those like Mary, single feels like who we are at our very core.

Some people are single by default or by defeat. That's not us. The single at heart are not single only because we "have issues" or because we are "too picky." We are not single just because we were unlucky in love or traumatized by previous romantic relationships. Single is not a phase for us. We will not outgrow it. Single life is not our Plan B. It is our first and best choice.

Single can be defined either legally or socially. You are officially, legally single if you are not married. You can be in a long-term, committed romantic relationship with someone you've been living with for decades, but if you never made it official, you are still legally single. You would not be socially single though. Socially single people do not have a serious romantic partner. They are the solo singles, single both legally and socially.

The "at heart" part of single at heart suggests a passion for single life, and an authenticity. It is also a door that opens a bit, to let in a few people who don't fit anyone's definition of single, but who, at heart, feel that single is who they really are. They are the people who are married or in a serious romantic relationship who yearn to be single, but do not want to hurt their partner by leaving. They also include people who have romantic partners they don't want to leave, but who insist that, at heart, they are single. As you will see, their relationships are not very conventional ones. They try to incorporate into their lives what the uncoupled single at heart find so dear, such as generous servings of solitude and boatloads of freedom.

Do You Qualify as Single at Heart?

The best way to know whether you are single at heart is to read the stories I'm sharing in this book of the people who already know that they qualify, and my discussions of the meaning of their experiences. The more you identify with those stories, the more likely you are to be single at heart. The more you *wish* you could be like them, the more likely it is that if you really gave single life a chance, you might like it more than you ever dreamed you could. Some people are like a woman I heard from during the pandemic, who desperately sought romantic coupling her whole life until she finally spent time on her own during the pandemic and discovered that she loved it.

Another way to get a sense of whether you are single at heart is to take the quiz at the end of this chapter. The quiz begins with fourteen questions. Then, participants are told, "If you are single at heart, single life suits you. You are not single because you have 'issues' or just haven't found a partner yet. Instead, living single is a way for you to lead your most meaningful and authentic life. Even people who are not single may be single at heart. Do you think you are single at heart?" In response, participants could choose from four answers: Yes; In more than a few ways, yes, but not all; Maybe in a few ways, but mostly not; and No.

People who are most clearly single at heart answer "Yes" to the question of whether they think they are single at heart. They typically give the single at heart answer to all fourteen questions, or close to it. The people who are most clearly not single at heart answer "No" to that question. They answer very few questions the way someone who is single at heart would, typically between zero and four questions.

I consider myself deeply and unambivalently single at heart, but I would not have scored a perfect fourteen on the quiz. My downfall is the question, "Do you have a sense of personal mastery—a can-do attitude and a sense that you can do just about anything you set your mind to?" Eighty-six percent of people who are clearly single at heart answer yes to that question. With their can-do attitude, and without the temptation to rely on a romantic partner to do what they don't know how to do or don't like to do, they master a whole array of skills. That serves them well throughout their lives. I'm in the 14 percent of the single at heart who do not have a sense of personal mastery. I don't think I can do just about anything I set my mind to; what's more, if it is something that doesn't interest me, I don't even want to try to learn it. In high school, for example, I very nearly failed a mechanical aptitude test. If I were married, I'd be shamelessly dependent on my spouse to do whatever I didn't like doing and I would have even fewer skills than I have now.

Of all the people who had taken the single at heart quiz by the time I analyzed the data for this book—nearly nine thousand people from more than one hundred nations—29 percent scored as clearly single at heart. Because the people who took the quiz were those who learned about it and were interested in it, and not a representative sample of the adults in the US or any other nation, the findings do not necessarily mean that 29 percent of all adults are single at heart.

In other research, representative national samples of German adults, eighteen and older, have been asked to indicate the extent of their agreement with the statement, "I would like to have a partner," on a five-point scale. Hebrew University sociologist Elyakim Kislev looked at the responses of the solo single people: they were not married, not cohabiting with a romantic partner, and did not have a romantic partner who lived elsewhere.[43] Some had never married, and others were divorced. More than fifty-six hundred participants fit those criteria. Overall, 21 percent of them said that they did not want a partner, choosing either the most definitive no ("not at all") or the next most definitive option. The people who were divorced were even more likely to say that they did not want a partner than the people who had never been married, 27 percent compared to 19 percent.

Not everyone who does not want a partner is single at heart. Some, for example, may be fed up with coupled life rather than enthralled by single life. Nonetheless, the results of the German survey and my own single at heart survey both suggest the same thing: substantial numbers of people just don't want to be coupled. Even as the over-the-top celebration of marriage, weddings, and coupling that I call "matrimania" continues to run wild, and even as many countries around the world continue to respect, value, and advantage people who are coupled over those who are single in their laws, policies, and practices, and in everyday social interactions, at least one in five single people in Germany, and probably in many other nations as well, are just saying "no thanks."

Our Joyful Lives

I always lived my most fulfilling, creative, happy, exciting life as a single.
—Eva (forty-four, London, England)

In describing single life in such exuberant terms, Eva speaks for many of us. In fact, if you want to answer just one question from the single at heart quiz, instead of all fourteen, to know if you are likely to be single at heart, it would be this one: "When you think about all the potential joys of single life, what do you conclude?" Of those who are clearly single at heart, 96 percent answer, "Sounds great!" Of those who are clearly not single at heart, only 7 percent think that single life sounds great.

We who are single at heart revel in our single life and all it has to offer. It's a delicious experience we get to savor every day. Sally, a forty-five-year-old from Austria, said, "Singledom is very much a state I enjoy and relish. I love to live alone, spend time alone, travel alone, and do things alone. I do not feel I am missing something or someone but feel happy and complete as an individual."

People who are powerfully drawn to single life, but who are currently in a romantic relationship, often find themselves yearning for their single lives. Sally shared, "I have enjoyed relationships when I have been in them but ultimately I felt a need to be on my own again and I never wanted to live with anyone." A man told me he was in a relationship with "a very nice guy," but added, "I have basically daydreamt about my solo life every day." A woman married to a man said, "More and more often, I fantasize about being alone again. Being free."

When social psychologist Wendy Morris and I studied stereotypes of single people, we found what we expected: people think single people are not as happy as married people.[44] They also think that single people become even more unhappy as they grow older. The single at heart defy those stereotypes. Over the course of their adult life, the more single people embrace their single lives, the more satisfied they feel. That's not just what I learned from the people who shared their life stories with me; it is also the conclusion of a study of more than seventeen thousand Germans, eighteen and older, who reported the degree to which they were pining for a partner, and their satisfaction with their lives, over and over again, for up to ten years.[45] Single people who are not trying to unsingle themselves are leading the life they want, and it just keeps getting better.

None of this means that we are happy all the time. No one is. But we are happy that we get to be single. We are grateful for our single lives in the best of times, and we are grateful even in the worst of times. When life taunts us with some of the most threatening experiences imaginable, we remain undeterred. The pandemic did not send us fleeing into the arms of a romantic partner. I live in Southern California, a land of wildfires. When a particularly ferocious fire came barreling toward my home and my phone blared with the warning that I had to evacuate immediately, I did not wish I had a romantic partner at my side. Kristin, age fifty-five, of Bellingham, Washington, who I'll talk more about later, faced the ultimate challenge. A car swerved into her as she was bicycling, leaving her mangled and barely breathing. She knew in those moments after she was hit that they could be her last, but she did not wish that she had stayed married. We really aren't just fooling ourselves about loving our single lives.

Because we who are single at heart love our single lives and don't want to ever unsingle ourselves, we are spared from some of the most painful emotions experienced by single people who really don't want to be single. One such emotion is the "ambiguous loss" of yearning to find a lifelong romantic partner, but not knowing whether that will ever happen. Karen Gail Lewis, author of *With or Without a Man*, defined that as "a loss for which there is no resolution," making it difficult to move on.[46] "Dear Therapist," an advice column, described it as "ambiguous grief—the intangible loss, the not knowing, the toggling between hope one minute and sadness the next."[47] It is hard for people struggling with that ambiguity to invest in their single lives and feel joyful about being single the way the single at heart do.

The single at heart are not spared from getting pitied. To be any kind of single person is to be at risk of being pitied. Sure, there are acknowledgments of strong, confident, happy single people in the media these days—I've done my share to encourage that—and yet the pity parties continue, mostly unabated.

To pity someone who is single at heart is to get our emotional profile all wrong. We know the feeling rules that tell us how we are supposed to experience things. But that's not how it works for us. One rule about feelings is that adults—women, especially—should feel badly when a younger sibling marries before they do. I was happy for my younger brother when he got married. I love him and his wife. Marriage is what he wanted. It is not what I wanted, and it is not what I ever wanted. Why would I feel bad about not having something I don't want? Lily, a thirty-six-year-old from West Virginia, put it this way: "When my brother got married, I was happy for him but I was detached from the whole ceremony. I didn't think, *Wow, I can't wait until I find someone and get married.*"

You can be single at heart and still be happy for people who are married. Single at heart is about being happily single. It is not about being anti-coupling or anti-marriage, though those attitudes are not disqualifying. I'm against using legal marriage as a criterion for access to special benefits and protections, as happens in the US, but for me, that's something different from being against romantic coupling.

My older brother is married. He and his wife live nearly two thousand miles away, but we visit each other and stay in touch. I'm the last person in the world who would know what goes on inside anyone's marriage, but they seem to have a very nice relationship, easy and loving. They've traveled the world together. They've gone to some fabulous restaurants. Stuck at home during the pandemic, they Zoomed into wine and cheese tastings hosted by the iconic New Orleans restaurant, Commander's Palace.

I'm happy for them too. I love them. And I'm not envious. I don't want to be part of a couple, not even an awesome one. If I were traveling the world with someone, I'd want my own room. I'd want to go off on my own some of the time. Maybe a lot of the time. I have had plenty of marvelous meals with friends and relatives, and I enjoyed every moment. When those dinner companions included couples, I have always been so very happy that I wasn't them. At the end of the evening, they went home together; I got to go home and be alone.

Another emotion rule that is routinely violated by people who are single at heart is how we feel if we get into a romantic relationship and it ends. We know that the break up of a serious relationship is supposed to be devastating. Maybe we even have friends or relatives who couldn't get out of bed for days after one. We who are single at heart sometimes also experience sadness and pain if a meaningful romantic relationship ends. But we experience something else too, sometimes much more strongly: relief. It feels good to return to the life that feels natural and comfortable for us, our single life. In the single at heart quiz, 84 percent of the single at heart reported feeling relief if they were in a romantic relationship that ended, compared to just 12 percent of people who are not single at heart.

We who are single at heart also break the rules about the things that are supposed to scare us. We are unafraid of loneliness because we are not very susceptible to it. We are unafraid of spending time alone, living alone, coming home to an empty home, going to bed alone, or waking up alone. We are unafraid of dining alone, traveling alone, or spending holidays and vacations alone. Most of us are unafraid of growing old alone, and yes, we are even unafraid of dying alone. Most importantly, most fundamentally, we are unafraid of being single. We *love* being single.

That's one of our superpowers. Because we are unafraid of being single, we get to invest joyfully and unreservedly in our single lives. We are spared from ruminating about what we might be missing, plotting ways to find The One, sinking time and money into the search, and presenting ourselves in ways we think will be most appealing to a potential partner.

A whole program of psychological research has explored the implications of being afraid of being single. Psychologist Stephanie Spielmann and her colleagues when she was at the University of Toronto created a scale to measure that fear, with items such as "I feel anxious when I think about being single forever" and "If I end up alone in life, I will probably feel that there is something wrong with me."[48] I'm more interested in the people who are *unafraid* of being single, the ones who disagree with those kinds of statements. They don't feel anxious or deficient when they think about staying single. Their psychological profiles are impressive. The fearlessly single are shown to be less likely to feel lonely and less likely to be depressed. They are also less neurotic and more open to new experiences.

Not everyone who is unafraid of being single is single at heart. Some people are unafraid of being single but are still interested in romantic coupling. Those people have standards.[49] They are not running away from single life toward anyone who will have them. Shown online profiles of potential dating partners, they are discriminating. They are mostly interested in people who seem caring and responsive. In contrast, people who are afraid of being single show almost as much interest in self-centered people. In speed dating events, people who are unafraid of being single give out their contact data to fewer people. When they do become romantically involved, they are less likely to feel needy and dependent. For example, they typically disagree with the statement, "If I couldn't be in this relationship, I would lose an important part of myself." They are also more likely to break off an unsatisfying romantic relationship than people who are afraid of being single.

People who are unafraid of being single also navigate the end of romantic relationships more skillfully, the research shows.[50] In the immediate aftermath, they are less likely to try to get back in touch with their ex, and they experience less yearning for their ex. Long after the breakup, people who are afraid of being single are still pining for their partner; those who are unafraid usually are not.

Just because the single at heart are unafraid of being single, that doesn't mean we have no fears at all. I live in fear that my computer will crash. I worry that the cost of living in my spectacularly beautiful Southern California town will eventually exceed my means. I'm scared that my health will someday fail so catastrophically that I will no longer be able live alone and care for myself. That last one is not a fear of being single, it is a fear of not being able to live my life as I wish to live it, independently in a place of my own.

In the chapter "Domestic Gulags" in her book *Against Love*, Laura Kipnis offers a sampling of the answers she got to the question, "What can't you do because you're in a couple?": "You can't leave the house without saying where you are going . . . you can't go to parties alone . . . you can't be a slob . . . you can't leave the dishes for later . . . you can't leave the bathroom door open . . . you can't watch soap operas without getting made fun of . . . you can't eat what you want."[51] It goes on like that for eight pages.

When a trio of social scientists studied a similar dynamic more systematically, they also found that being with a romantic partner can be draining.[52] In the study, more than three hundred coupled people, ranging in age from nineteen to ninety-two, described who they were with and how they were feeling on at least two occasions. Being with their partner did not protect them from feeling frustrated, worried, sad, or angry. In fact, except for the people who stood out from the rest in consistently describing their relationship in the most positive ways, the participants experienced more of those negative feelings when they were with their partner than when their partner was not around.

When I hear from people who want to stay single, sometimes they tell me stories about the things they were not allowed to do when they were in a romantic relationship, or how they felt more self-conscious or more wary or more inadequate or more miserable when their partner was around than when they were alone or with friends. They chafe at what romantic partnering meant to them, and they don't want to go back to that ever again.

Some women tell me they got tired of doing more than their fair share of the dishes and the laundry and the caretaking and organizing outings and remembering everyone's birthday. Some men tell me they felt suffocated.

I also hear from people who have trust issues, or who have parents who criticized them relentlessly when they were children and then never stopped. Some confide their history of emotional problems. Some report that they have never seen a committed relationship they would want for themselves; their parents were not good role models, and neither was anyone else.

I listen to them with great interest; but if their only reasons for wanting to stay single are negative ones, they are not single at heart. We who are single at heart love being single, and not because we are running away from coupled life or nursing old wounds; we are leaping into the arms of our single life because of the opportunities it offers for us to flourish.

What about the people who thrive when they are single but who also have had troubling experiences? Holly, who is thirty-four and from the Washington, DC, area believes she is single at heart. "I'm good on my own," she told me. "I'm very independent, love to do my own thing, do quick solo weekend trips, go to dinner on my own, and have an active social life."

She's worried, though, that she may identify as single at heart for the wrong reasons, and that's why she wrote to me. She struggled with obsessive-compulsive disorder (OCD) in her childhood and through her twenties. She had some decent experiences when dating, but also some traumatizing ones.

Holly is happily single, but other people keep telling her that what she's experiencing isn't really happiness, and that she's in denial. They tell her she just hasn't met the right person yet. They pathologize her, proclaiming that she is afraid of intimacy. And sometimes she doubts herself. She wonders whether her struggles with OCD make her "closed off to romantic relationships." She's concerned that maybe she just hasn't tried hard enough at dating.

I told Holly that I don't think it matters at all if her experiences with dating were disastrous or delightful. It doesn't matter if she had OCD or has been a paragon of mental health. We who are single at heart are not defined or motivated by what we have left behind. If Holly wanted to be single only as an escape from her painful dating experiences, or solely as a way of dodging anything else she did not like, then she would not be single at heart. But Holly, who is very independent, who happily travels on her own and goes out to dinner on her own and also has an active social life, is really good at single life. She should be congratulating herself, and her friends should look up to her.

If you are single, you may recognize what has happened to Holly—she has gotten the singles treatment. Her own feelings of happiness have not been taken at face value; they have been doubted and examined and turned against her.

I encouraged Holly to do something I advise throughout this book: flip the script. Imagine asking married people if they really are happily married or if they are just fooling themselves. Imagine speculating that the real reason they are married is that they never learned to stand on their own two feet. Maybe some pathology is in play—they are just too needy and dependent to be single.

Holly worried that she didn't try hard enough at dating. But why aren't coupled people concerned that they may not have tried hard enough to live single?

I don't think anyone, coupled or single, should be treated in disrespectful ways. Coupled people typically are not. It is the single people, especially those who love their single lives, who are put on the defensive. They shouldn't be.

Our Psychologically Rich Lives

I was raised by society to dream of my wedding,
but I wish I had been dreaming of my life.[53]
—Tracee Ellis Ross

"You complete me," Tom Cruise said to Renée Zellweger in a scene from *Jerry Maguire* that remains iconic more than a quarter-century later. You can mock the sentiment, but many people believe it with all their heart. Without a romantic partner—just the right romantic partner—they feel incomplete and shrunken, like something is missing.

Not the single at heart. For us it is single life that is expansive, that affords us a whole wide world of possibilities. If we settled for a life of conventional marriage or long-term romantic coupling, our lives would feel smaller. That, to us, would be a lesser life. That's not how everyone experiences coupled life, of course, but it is how we do.

Our lives feel full of possibilities when we can open our arms to as many or as few people as we like, with no pressure to choose one person and prioritize that person above all others. Our lives feel full of potential when we can afford ourselves the solitude we find so enriching and restorative. Our lives feel expansive when we can use our freedom to pursue our passions, to do work we find meaningful, or to be there for the people who mean the most to us. Our lives feel fulfilling when we can create homes that are our sanctuaries in places where we love to live.

Sara Braca, author of *When the Church Burns Down, Cancel the Wedding*, told me that partnered people often get it wrong when they ask her about her personal life. "The underlying assumption always seems to be that I'm looking for love, but I'm really looking for life!"

When people who are single at heart shared their life stories with me, one after another effused about the variety of experiences their single lives offered them. Sally (forty-five, Austria) said, "My life is rich, full, varied, and interesting." Acadia of Melbourne, Australia, said, "I already feel like at thirty-six I've done so much more than I expected to do. I thought all I could do is work a boring job, get married, and have children. It turns out life—including work—is *so much better* than that and has *so* many more opportunities."

Mary (thirty-three, Buffalo, New York) said, "I see life as one big opportunity to learn, do, see, and evolve as much as I can. I welcome new experiences." What she, Sally, Acadia, and others were describing was not just a joyful life, but a psychologically rich one.

To many people all around the world, a good life is a happy life. The social scientists Shigehiro Oishi of the University of Virginia and Erin C. Westgate of the University of Florida asked people in nine nations—Angola, Germany, India, Japan, Norway, Portugal, Singapore, South Korea, and the United States—to describe their ideal life.[54] A happy life was the most popular choice in every nation. A meaningful life was also highly valued. Others described their ideal life as a psychologically rich life, one that was eventful and full of interesting and unique experiences. In each nation, at least 7 percent, and as many as 17 percent, of respondents said that if they had to choose just one kind of life, they would want the psychologically rich life, even at the expense of a happy life and a meaningful life.

Fortunately it is not necessary to choose just one. Each offers something different. A happy life includes comfort, joy, and security. A meaningful life is a life of significance and purpose. A psychologically rich life, Oishi and Westgate explain, is "characterized by a variety of interesting and perspective-changing experiences," and people who lead psychologically rich lives are rewarded with the wisdom that comes from their diverse experiences.[55]

On their deathbeds, a person who led a happy life might say, "I had fun!" whereas a person who had a meaningful life would think, *I made a difference!* The parting thoughts of the person who led a psychologically rich life would be, *What a journey!*

People who are single at heart experience their single lives as joyful. They value meaningfulness too. In the quiz, for example, people who are single at heart are more likely than those who are not single at heart to say that they would choose meaningful work over work that paid a lot if they could not have both. But it may be the psychological richness of their lives that is most distinctive.

Oishi and Westgate suggest something similar:

> According to Kierkegaard [the Danish theologian], a married person with a secure, well-respected job and children may have a happy and (in many respects) meaningful life, but not necessarily a life rich in diverse perspective-changing experiences. Although most people choose such a conventional, secure, and well-respected life, others . . . choose the esthetic wanderer's life instead—unconventional, unstable, and uncompromising.[56]

People who lead psychologically rich lives, Oishi and Westgate found, are curious and open-minded. They have unconventional attitudes, they experience personal growth, and they don't want to socialize with the same person all the time. The single at heart share all of those characteristics. In the quiz, for example, they are especially likely to say that they do not want a romantic partner to be the one most important person in their lives and they also do not like the idea of having one person who is their "plus-one" for just about every occasion. They prefer to have more options, more variety, and more interpersonal richness.

A study of US adults at midlife compared people who stayed single with those who stayed married over a five-year period. The single people were more likely to agree with statements such as "For me, life has been a continuous process of learning, change, and growth." The married people more often endorsed other kinds of sentiments, such as, "I gave up trying to make big improvements in my life a long time ago."[57]

The variety of unique and interesting experiences that make a life psychologically rich do not all have to be joyful ones. Experiences that are challenging or even tragic can add psychological richness to life. Widowhood, for example, can be devastating, but it can also change a person's perspective in a way that is psychologically enriching.

David, a sixty-five-year-old in Austin, Texas, has had a successful career in broadcasting, animation, and writing original musical scores. He is also an avid traveler whose adventures have included working with medicine people in the Amazon and climbing the Matterhorn in Switzerland. When he learned about the research on psychologically rich lives, he told me:

> The psychologically rich life is just exactly what I desire for myself and what I have pursued from the beginning, even when I did not know that this was what I was doing. I consider myself to be one of the most fortunate people on the planet. Though I've had my share of negative and hurtful challenges, I've also had so many wonderful true adventures

and learning experiences, most of which I have initiated on purpose. It's good to be rich, they say, and though I haven't much money, I am richer than most people ever get to be, just from the direction I've pointed myself. I'm paid with the currency of the psychologically rich life: experiences that change me, and a true form of wisdom.

People leading psychologically rich lives are often liberal. "Those leading happy and/or meaningful lives tend to prefer to maintain social order and the status quo," Oishi and Westgate note, "whereas those leading psychologically rich lives seem to embrace social change."[58] People who are single at heart can be found across the political spectrum, but they too are more often liberal than conservative, analyses of the quiz data showed.

Our Authentic Lives

I feel like my most authentic self when I'm single.
—Evan (forty, San Francisco, California)

Authenticity is at the core of what it means to be single at heart. Single is who we really are. To us, single life feels natural and comfortable. To live some other way would feel forced. Some of us have tried to live the coupled life that is expected of us. It never felt right, not even with partners we truly loved and who loved us back. At best, we often felt empty and bored, like we were just going through the motions; at worst, we felt fraudulent and miserable. When people who are single at heart describe their lives, they use the language of authenticity.

To Acadia (thirty-six, Melbourne, Australia), the best thing about being single is "the freedom to be my true, authentic self." Sally (forty-five, Austria) said that being single "is my natural and preferred state. Not a lack of options but a choice to live my life on my terms." Liz, age sixty, of Washington, DC, said, "I believe I am living the life I was meant to have."

Scholars who study our deepest needs and motives see authenticity as essential to human flourishing.[59] If we pursue goals that do not reflect who we really are, what we care about, and what we are good at, then even if we achieve our goals, we are not going to be truly happy or fulfilled. That dynamic is evident in the stories of people who are single at heart who tried, sometimes repeatedly, to live the coupled life they thought they were supposed to live, only to feel dissatisfied every time. Only when they understood themselves as single at heart and embraced single life did they feel like they were coming home to their true self.

For her master's thesis at New Mexico State University, Kristen M. Bernhardt interviewed twenty-five people she called "agentically single."[60] I think of them as cousins of the single at heart: not looking for a lifelong monogamous partner at the time of the interview, but not necessarily ruling that out in the future. Among the participants in Bernhardt's research were people who had been in long-term monogamous coupled relationships in the past but realized they would prefer to be free agents. People who had never been married or coupled, including some who were asexual and/or aromantic, were also part of the project, as were solo polyamorous people who may or may not have been in one or more relationships, both sexual and nonsexual. What all of those agentically single people had in common, Bernhardt said, was "a sense of pride and self-worth in having overcome past insecurities and living their lives as they feel they are meant to be lived. They were happy because they were living authentically."

Anyone of any relationship status can live authentically. People who are single at heart, though, who are bucking powerful social norms, are especially likely to think deeply about who they really are and what they really want. The prevailing presumption about how we are supposed to want to live was defined by philosophy professor Elizabeth Brake as amatonormativity, "the assumption that a central, exclusive, amorous relationship is normal for humans, in that it is a universally shared goal, and that such a relationship is normative, in the sense that it *should* be aimed at in preference to other relationship types."[61] The single at heart reject that, as does Brake. In the quiz, 86 percent of the single at heart, compared to just 8 percent of those who are not single at heart, said they were uninterested in searching for a romantic partner. We are amatonormativity busters.

In her popular essay on the rise of the "alpha single," people who don't want to forsake their independence for the sake of being coupled, Hattie Crisell, age thirty-four, shares that she had been in many romantic relationships over the years. In the most recent serious one, she tried hard to compromise on many matters, hoping that would be the ticket to relationship staying power. "What I could no longer compromise on in the end," she wrote, "was happiness, or my sense of who I was, which I could feel slipping away. Even though we loved each other, that wasn't enough to keep up the exhausting contortions of trying to make it work."[62]

People who are single at heart and who had romantic relationships have often had that feeling that they are drifting away from the person they really are. In their experiences, that sense of inauthenticity in coupled relationships was not something that happened only with particular partners who weren't a good fit. Instead, it was something about romantic relationships more generally. Craig, age forty-one, of Newport News, Virginia, said, "I always feel more 'natural' when I'm single as opposed to when I'm in relationships."

Eva (forty-four, London, England) said, "I fell into the pressure and tried to date, even have a romantic relationship, but it always felt like the wrong size of shoes, just uncomfortable."

People whose best life is single life, and who free themselves from the pressures to live a conventional coupled life, are no longer at war with themselves. By living authentically, they become better friends, better confidants, and, if it interests them, better lovers. They are able to think more clearly and immerse themselves in their passions unreservedly.

In choosing to embrace single life, they also spare potential romantic partners frustration. In an essay, Vera, age fifty-two, wrote, "I stopped dating and I couldn't be happier. . . . Deep down, I entered some relationships to stave off loneliness or because it was something that I was expected to do. The immense harm that I caused myself and some of the men I dated because I didn't behave as my authentic self causes me great pain."[63] To live single instead of drawing another person into a coupled life you don't really want is an act of generosity and love.

Many of the People Living Joyful, Psychologically Rich, Authentic Single Lives Are Men

In 1898 the *Atlantic Monthly* published a lengthy profile of the person who may well be the most famous single man you have never heard of.[64] Henry Crabb Robinson was a beloved figure in the literary circles of nineteenth century London. He hosted Sunday breakfasts at his home and befriended scores of literary luminaries.

Crabb Robinson was a passionate reader and critic, and a prolific writer of letters and diaries. When he found a poem he loved, he wanted his friends to know about it. "He championed Wordsworth's poetry at a time when champions were few and not influential," Leon H. Vincent, the author of the profile, noted. Goethe, who described him as "a kind of missionary of English literature," said that Crabb Robinson read poems to him and his daughter.[65]

Born in 1775, when the life expectancy of a white man was about thirty-eight years, Crabb Robinson lived to be ninety-two. In his later years, he spent Christmas at the home of Wordsworth, where "his presence was considered essential to the sober merrymaking of the household there. They had a family saying, 'No Crabb, no Christmas.'"[66]

Crabb Robinson traveled extensively and walked for many miles throughout Germany, Wales, Switzerland, and Italy, sometimes with friends. He was a barrister and the first foreign correspondent for *The Times* of

London. He had a hand in the founding of the University of London and was involved in an antislavery campaign. What merited a place on his tombstone, though, were the names of eight of his friends, including Wordsworth, Goethe, Blake, and Coleridge.

"This man had a brilliant career," wrote Vincent. "He lived long, which gave him time to see many things; he had good health, which enabled him to enjoy what he saw. Life tasted sweet to him up to the last day, and almost to the last hour. His wholesome curiosity about good books and good people never failed . . . there were few things worth knowing of which he did not know something, and few people worth cultivating whom he had not cultivated."[67] The profile ended with this sentence: "He was a successful bachelor and a good man."[68]

Henry Crabb Robinson, a lifelong single man, had a joyful and psychologically rich life. My guess is that he also had an authentic single life. The *Atlantic Monthly*, though, was not celebrating Crabb Robinson as an example of a whole category of single men who were flourishing. Instead he was cast as a remarkable exception. "More interest should be taken in bachelors," the magazine explained in a quote pulled from Vincent's article. "Their need is greater, and their condition really deplorable. It is a misfortune to be unhappily married, but it comes near to being a disgrace not to be married at all."[69]

More than a century later, I think single men are still more often demeaned than respected. They are stereotyped as slobs or playboys, perverts or mama's boys, perpetual children living in their parents' basements. Some contribute to their own marginalization by identifying as "incels," involuntarily celibate men, and embracing hostile and misogynistic attitudes. The social sciences have not always been flattering either. Studies have shown that on average it is women, more than men, who seem to take to single life.[70] They like it better. They like their solitude more. They spend more time pursuing their interests. They are more likely to have fulfilling friendships— they are good at connecting and staying connected with the people who matter to them. Domestic chores are not a challenge; they've often been raised to know how to cook and clean. Single women who were previously married to a man often express relief at no longer doing more than their share of those tasks and of caretaking too.

For people of every gender, "happily ever after" is just a fairy tale. More than a dozen studies that followed the same people for years have shown that when couples move in together or when they marry, they do not become lastingly happier or healthier than they were when they were single.[71] Marriage does not magically transform them. Women and men are mostly the same in that regard. When there are differences, though, it is typically the men who are more likely to benefit from being married and the women who do better when they are single.[72] Once married, women are more likely to want out; in the US, more divorces are initiated by women than by men.[73] Once divorced or widowed, women are more likely to stay out; they remarry less often than men.[74]

Single women, though, hardly get a free ride. Discrepancies in pay, especially for women of color, make it more challenging for them to live on their own.[75] Women typically suffer greater financial losses after a divorce.[76] Unmarried women are often less financially secure than unmarried men as they head into retirement.[77] And social dynamics differ too. Single women more often feel pressure to answer for their uncoupled status.[78] They get labeled as spinsters, and despite efforts to reclaim the term, it still seems more demeaning than being called a bachelor.

Contemporary books, articles, essays, and blog posts about single life are overwhelmingly written for, by, and about single women. In a way, single women have more to prove. They are the ones who are believed to be yearning for romantic coupling, eager to build their lives around marriage, and bereft when that doesn't happen, no matter what the studies say. But even if their writings seem motivated by an attempt to justify a single status that should never be in need of justification, they can be affirming. In writing about their lives, single women are being heard. They are forcefully pushing back against all the narratives that belittle them.

Because women really do, on average, fare better than men when single, because more of them are writing about the joy they find in living single, and because men are less vocal in their rejection of the many stereotypes that disparage them, it is easy to imagine that many more women than men are single at heart. That's not, however, what I found when I analyzed the data from the single at heart quiz. Of all the men who took the quiz, 34 percent of them qualified as clearly single at heart, compared to 27 percent of the women. These are the people who answered "Yes" to the question at the end of the quiz about whether they think they are single at heart, meaning that "living single is a way for you to lead your most meaningful and authentic life." They typically answered all fourteen of the questions, or thirteen of the fourteen questions, in the single at heart direction. When I looked at the people who said that they were mostly single at heart, and who typically answered between nine and twelve of the fourteen questions in the single at heart direction, I again found that a greater proportion of the men than of the women qualified.

Men, it seems, are at least as likely as women, and probably even more likely, to be powerfully drawn to single life. These men find single life to be joyful and psychologically rich; it is how they live most authentically. Like the women who flourish when single, they too savor the time they have to themselves rather than fearing it. They cherish their freedom to build their best life, whether that is a life of adventure, meaningful work, devotion to a cause, caring for people in need, or anything else they find fulfilling. They learn the skills that have been stereotyped as women's work, such as creating and managing a home, and attending to the people who matter to them.

In a guest post for my "Living Single" blog on the *Psychology Today* website, Lucas Bradley, then age thirty-seven, of Loves Park, Illinois, described the Deliberately Single Man:

> Who is the Deliberately Single Man? He cultivates the histor-
> ically "feminine" qualities of domestic, social, and emotion-
> al literacy in order to live a connected and dignified life. For
> example, domestically, he learns to plan and make healthy

meals and is able to develop an aesthetic for his living space that suits his tastes. Socially, he works to maintain ties with those he is close to by initiating get-togethers and remembering birthdays and other milestones. Emotionally, he tries to stay curious and nonjudgmental about his thoughts and feelings and cultivate appropriate outlets for his emotions. The Deliberately Single Man also reimagines love in a way that empowers those he loves rather than limiting them with a set of Byzantine rules and expectations. He recognizes that romantic love is not the only road to wholeness and cultivates many other forms of love available to him. He realizes that his singlehood, far from being what's holding him back, can actually be the primary engine for his growth as a person.[79]

When Craig Wynne (forty-one, Newport News, Virginia) was eight, his best friend confided that what he wanted out of life was a wife, kids, and lots of sex. Craig aspired to something different: "I want to live in a house by myself and own a candy store." He still doesn't have that candy store, but he does have a place of his own and a sweet job that includes teaching students something they rarely learn about in college—sophisticated thinking about what it can mean to be single. He has been out front in getting the scholarly study of single people on the map. With Ketaki Chowkhani, age thirty-four, of Manipal, India, he organized the first global Singles Studies conference, and the two edited an anthology of papers from the conference.[80] He also wrote *How to Be a Happy Bachelor*, an affirming book for single men, full of tips for living a fulfilling single life, as well as some brilliant critiques of the misrepresentation of single people in popular culture.[81]

In 2015 I started the Facebook group the Community of Single People for people who want to savor their single lives rather than escape them. It has nothing to do with dating. As of early 2023, it had more than seventy-four hundred members from more than one hundred nations. Craig is one of the most involved participants, responsive to other members' questions and concerns, and regularly posting pictures of his "son" Chester (his cat). He has also taken the initiative to do what many craved when they joined the Community—he's arranged to meet other members in person for conversation, dining, hikes, and outings in and around the place where he lives and the places he visits.

In Kenya in 2021, the Saturday magazine of *Nation.Africa* posed this question: What happens to men who stay bachelors for a lifetime? One of the men interviewed for the article was a forty-seven-year-old businessman, Stephen Mutahi. Describing lifelong single men like himself, he said, "We are rich in friendship." He has traveled extensively, noting, "I have met many friends who I believe I would never have met if I was married or in a serious relationship."[82] When he socializes with women, he makes it clear that he is not interested in a romantic relationship. Like the men who identify as single at heart, Mutahi loves his space and values the freedom he has to arrange his everyday life as he sees fit.

Each of the men who shared their life stories with me is living their own version of the single at heart life. I'll tell you more about them throughout this book. What their stories reveal, together with the stories of other men thriving in their single lives, is that all those demeaning stereotypes don't define single men like them. Neither do the studies that average across all single men and proclaim that men typically are not doing all that well at living single. Today's men who are single at heart are not average or typical; they are exceptional. Like Henry Crabb Robinson, they are successful bachelors and good men.

THE QUIZ: ARE YOU SINGLE AT HEART?

1. **When you think about spending time alone, what thought comes to mind first?**
   A. "Ah, sweet solitude!"
   B. "Oh, no, I might be lonely!"

2. **How do you feel about searching for a long-term romantic partner?**
   A. Maybe it feels like something you "should" do, but you are not really all that interested.
   B. The process may or may not be exciting and fun, but a successful outcome would be great!

3. **If you were/are in a romantic relationship and it ended, how did/ would you feel?**
   A. Mostly sadness and pain.
   B. Some pain, but also relief. The thought of being your own complete person filled you with joy.

4. **When you are thinking about making a big change in your life, such as embarking on a new career or moving across the country, which do you prefer?**
   A. Making the decision with a partner, even if that means that you do not pursue your favorite option.
   B. Making the decision that feels right to you, without worrying about whether a partner would approve, or whether your decision might stand in the way of a partner's goals.

5. **Many couples expect to be each other's "plus-one" for just about every occasion. How do you feel about that?**

A. You prefer to have more options, sometimes attending events on your own, sometimes with other people, and sometimes just staying home when the event doesn't interest you.

B. You take comfort in having a person in your life who is obligated to be your plus-one when you want to go somewhere, even though you will be obligated to be your partner's plus-one at events that you might prefer to skip.

6. **Think about the possibility that when you go to sleep at night, there might not be anyone else in bed with you. How does that make you feel?**
   A. You would not like that.
   B. You are fine with that.

7. **Ideally who would be the most important adults in your life?**
   A. Your spouse (or long-term romantic partner) would be the most important person to you. Other people would be peripheral.

   B. You would not want a romantic partner to be the one most important person in your life. You might prefer to have a personal community comprised of a mix of people, such as friends, family, and coworkers. Or you might want to focus mostly on friends. The number of important people in your life, and how close you'd like to be to them, might be different at different times.

8. **When you are tempted to allow yourself your favorite indulgence, such as eating junk food or watching trashy TV, how do you feel?**
   A. Delighted to do exactly as you wish, with no one else around.
   B. You prefer to have a spouse at your side, either to join you in your sloth or badger you to exert more self-control.

9. **When you want to pursue lofty goals, such as eating right, getting lots of exercise, or reading inspiring books, which would you prefer?**
   A. Pursuing those plans on your own or with friends.
   B. Having a partner who will pursue those plans along with you, or provide an excuse to do something else instead.

10. **When you have had some minor mishap such as a fender bender, how do you feel?**
    A. You would be relieved not to have to explain to anyone else why you messed up.
    B. You want to have a partner to go home to and tell all about it.

11. **If you had to choose between meaningful work that did not pay much or uninspiring work that paid a lot, which would you pick?**
    A. The meaningful work that did not pay much.
    B. The uninspiring work that paid a lot.

12. **Do you have a sense of personal mastery—a can-do attitude and a sense that you can do just about anything you set your mind to?**
    A. No
    B. Yes

13. **Are you self-sufficient—do you like handling problems and challenges mostly on your own?**
    A. No
    B. Yes

14. **When you think about all of the potential joys of single life, what do you conclude?**

A. Sounds great!

B. You recognize the appeal, but coupling is so compelling to you that single life just doesn't compare.

15. **This quiz is a first step toward identifying people who are single at heart. If you are single at heart, single life suits you. You are not single because you have "issues" or just haven't found a partner yet. Instead, living single is a way for you to lead your most meaningful and authentic life. Even people who are not single may be single at heart. Do you think you are single at heart?**

- Yes
- In more than a few ways, yes, but not all
- Maybe in a few ways, but mostly not
- No

The people who took the quiz were also invited "to make suggestions or comments about any aspect of this survey or the topic of being single at heart."

Scoring Key: People who are single at heart typically choose these answers:

1. A
2. A
3. B
4. B
5. A
6. B
7. B
8. A
9. A
10. A
11. A
12. B

13. B

14. A

People who choose more of these answers are more likely to be single at heart.

In response to Question 15, "Do you think you are single at heart?":

- People who answer "Yes" typically score 13 or 14.
- People who respond "in more than a few ways" typically score between 9 and 12.
- People who respond "maybe in a few ways" typically score between 5 and 8.
- People who answer "No" typically score between 0 and 4.

2

The Pressures to Live a Coupled Life and How We Conquered Them

We who are single at heart love being single. To us, single life is liberating. But we are not immune from the relentless pressures to couple up. Those pressures got to some of us, and for way too long held us back from understanding that single life was our best life. Ultimately, in our own ways, each of us prevailed over the forces that keep so many people from recognizing the fulfillment and the power of a life uncoupled.

We Tried It All—Romantic Coupling, Marriage, Remarriage, and More

People who are single at heart have two big things going for them: they find single life deeply satisfying and they are not powerfully drawn to coupled life. Why, then, do some people who are so well suited to living single keep trying to make romantic coupling work, even after disappointing experiences?

We keep trying because we think that we just chose the wrong person. Or we weren't mature enough then, but now we are. Or we did not love ourselves enough to love someone else, and now we do. We keep trying because we are afraid that if we stay single, we will let our parents down. We keep trying because many of our friends have already headed down the path of romantic coupledom, and that makes it seem like we should too. We keep trying because the friends who included us when they were single no longer do so now that they are coupled, and that hurts. We keep trying because our steps toward success at romantic coupling are recognized and celebrated. Everyone is so happy for us when we are coupled! We get included in the Couples Club. That sort of validation can feel intoxicating.

We keep trying for pragmatic reasons, maybe because a partner is a ticket to good health insurance or all the other legal benefits and protections of marriage or the promise of a better life by way of a fiancée visa.

We keep trying because we so rarely find themes of glorious lifelong singlehood in novels, TV shows, movies, poems, or songs. It is as if only romantic coupling can be truly, deeply, enduringly fulfilling.

All of that, and so much more, seems like a lot to give up. But somehow, for us, the life of conventional romantic coupling just doesn't work. It is not fulfilling. It is not who we really are. When we are in a life organized around romantic coupling, we want out. We are never truly contented until we commit to our single lives and stop trying to unsingle ourselves.

Here are the stories of a few of us who have tried and tried again to love coupled life.

Jennifer, age forty-five, lives in Denver and has never been married. She is currently so happy being single that she has supplemented her corporate job with self-employment as a life coach, helping other singles thrive in their solo lives. She could have benefited from such a coach when she was younger. Here's her story in her own words:

> When I was twenty-two years old I began what would be a ten-year relationship with a man. We were happy. No big drama happened, we always got along well, and I did love him. And at eight years, we got engaged. We also happened to be living together.
>
> It was strange, but within about three months I began getting those feelings that I believe people refer to as cold feet. I quickly became uninterested in planning a wedding. And I started to think of all of the things I hadn't done with just me on my own, like live in a different city or take a job overseas. Also, I was starting to feel like the engagement and marriage were an ending . . . an ending of my own life, and it was giving me this feeling of hollowness and a sadness.

It was feeling like my life was over, and the life that was approaching (a married life) didn't bring me a sense of excitement or a lot to look forward to.

I was also always undecided on having children, and that wasn't changing either. There were plenty of people around me saying, "Oh, you just wait. By the time you get to thirty-two you'll want kids. Oh, just wait, thirty-seven, yep thirty-seven you'll really want kids and then there might not be a man around." Well, I wasn't changing my mind on that, and started to communicate that to him. He'd always say that we could do the things I wanted to do . . . take a job in another state, travel the world, live overseas even with kids. But here's the thing, I never saw myself doing those things with someone, like a husband and kids. I wanted to be free to move about life on my own, in my own way and on my own terms.

I ended the engagement when I was thirty-two years old, and I remember thinking to myself that I was going to take the remainder of my thirties to be on my own. And then I could meet someone in my early forties and be good with that. I dated here and there, but nothing amazing came my way that would change my plan. And again, when a relationship began to drift, I'd feel a sense of relief and renewal of me. Sometimes I think I kept dating as a "should," something I should still do. And each year I would think to myself, "Maybe this is the year that I'll be interested in meeting someone. Maybe this year I'll have the desire to date." But I never truly did.

Then, on my forty-forth birthday, I remember thinking that I didn't have to think that way anymore. I didn't have to wonder when I'll be interested in a relationship. And I remember thinking that I loved my life how it's been: me single and on my own. And that I was so joyful and had so much gratitude for my life.

Jennifer gave conventional coupled life every possible chance. She met someone she loved. She got engaged. Her fiancé loved her so much that he reassured her that she could still do all the things she was worried about missing if she married him. When she broke up with him, she allowed herself about a decade to live on her own before returning to the project of finding a romantic partner. Maybe she thought she'd get it out of her system, that urge to be on her own. But nothing worked. Single life was not something she could get out of her system. It was her system.

The choice to break off the engagement was the right one for Jennifer. It is often the right one for women who have cold feet as the day of their wedding approaches. Research shows that if they go ahead and marry, they are more likely to divorce than women who don't have cold feet, and if they stay married, they end up less satisfied with their relationship.[83]

Other people who are single at heart have gone through with their marriages, even when their misgivings ran as deep as Jennifer's were. Some married more than once. They followed the conventional wisdom that maintains that it is romantic partnering that brings happiness. No one ever says, "You deserve to be happy—stay single." And so, when people who are single at heart get married and end up as miserable as they thought they would be, sometimes they just try again.

That's what happened to Sophia, a fifty-seven-year-old science editor and writer. She raised three children and was living alone on a boat in a marina in England when she told me about her life. Here's what she shared:

> I thought I was supposed to get married. I remember think-
> ing to myself when I was engaged that I really needed to have
> something else in my life because marriage was not going to
> make me happy. How scary (or stupid) that I was so aware of
> how little I wanted it, and yet I still went through with it!

I was so deliriously happy after my two divorces (particularly the second one) that it never occurred to me to try for that again. After three or so years of singleness I tried dating, but I was going through the motions. I was really happy by myself. It was a good exercise in proving to me that I really had no interest in a romantic relationship.

I've been single for thirteen years, and I have never been happier. Ever. I'm having a great life, and I only wish I had started this journey with myself much sooner.

These days, Sophia said, "I want to live freely and from my heart, rather than following societal rules that I had no part in creating."

For some who are single at heart, having the experience of marriage feels right, even if the marriage ends in divorce. It affirms their understanding of themselves as single at heart in a way that does not seem possible otherwise. That's the perspective of David (sixty-five, Austin, Texas). He has had a long successful career in broadcasting and other creative arts and describes himself as "a creative introvert who is happily single." Here's David's story:

It was only in my late thirties and just into my early forties that I realized that time was getting away, and I felt pressured in my own mind to meet someone for marriage. I joined several different commercial dating services and worked my way through that quite artificial and forced process. It was really emotionally difficult and mostly disheartening. At last, however, I did connect with one woman who was intellectual, had many similar interests, had the same type of humor with a penchant for puns as myself, etc. We dated and the pressure built for me to propose, which I decided to do in 1995.

I do believe now that marriage was a good and a necessary experience for both of us. Without it I would have always wondered about what I had missed or failed to do in life. We had what I would call a very good and decent "marriage of friends," which we actually were and still are. At our older ages when we married (I was forty-two), we decided not to try to have children.

Our life paths were different, though, and many practical things caused those paths to diverge. I still wanted and needed to be my solo self, doing my solo things. I began to feel constricted and smothered by my obligation and she also had issues with it. We divorced, amicably, after nine years. I am extremely thankful and glad that we have maintained our real friendship ever since then.

When I was considering the divorce, I looked back at my previous unmarried life and one thing stood out to me. I knew that regardless of the "I should be married by now" religious/psychological/cultural overlay, I had been truly happy as a single man. When I made that critical decision to leave the marriage and move on with my own life as a reborn single man, it was an electric and amazing feeling of new freedom. It was like finding myself all over again, but with a clean slate ahead for anything I wanted to make out of life. I have not lost that powerful sense of thrill in the many years since, and I know it now for what it is: my authentic self as a single at heart person.

Kristin (fifty-five, Bellingham, Washington) told me: "I never dreamed of a wedding day. I dreamed of living alone." Kristin's road to living the single at heart life, though, wound through marriage to a man, divorce, and coming out as a lesbian.

I remember my friends systematically abandoning me in my teens for (yuck) boys. I started dating simply because there weren't any girls around to hang out with anymore. I hated it, but still felt validated when I had a date. Eventually I married a man who didn't expect me to wear itchy or demeaning things to bed. The night before I got married, I felt so sad, and later, when I heard Carly Simon's song "You Want to Marry Me" [officially titled "That's the Way I've Always Heard It Should Be"], I bawled for hours because it so perfectly captured that feeling I had [that I should do what was expected of me].

I stuck with the marriage longer than I should have, and I was able to because he traveled so much for business, we were mostly LAT [living apart together]. During that time I explored relationships with women and thought that was where I belonged. When Kenn was relentlessly home for two years, I snapped and left, and moved to this town because of its thriving lesbian scene.

I remember, though, after a date with a woman thirteen years ago, thinking, *I hate dating no matter who it's with*, and decided not to do it anymore. Then I discovered that there are people who love being single and realized it was a whole thing, that I could come out again as single at heart.

In the quiz, 84 percent of the single at heart who had been in a romantic relationship said that when such a relationship ended, they may have felt some pain, but they also felt relieved. Only 12 percent of the people who were not single at heart felt relieved. Now that I have heard so many of the life stories of people who are single at heart, I realize that experiencing that relief is part of a broader process of understanding ourselves. At some point, people who are single at heart and who have pursued romantic relationships don't just feel relieved that a particular relationship has ended; they realize that they don't want any romantic relationship to be the center of their lives ever again. That's an even bigger relief.

Mary (thirty-three, Buffalo, New York) has always enjoyed her own company best. "Even when I was a child, I was always wandering off to play by myself. For as long as I can remember, I had an understanding of myself as an autonomous unit, not some half of a whole, not part of a family."

That never changed, but her feelings about it did. In her early adult years, she started feeling ashamed of her single at heart nature. She tried hard to conform. She had two serious romantic relationships, and even found them somewhat intriguing at first. But, she added, "I felt like I couldn't be the best version of myself while I was in them." Mary did not fault her partners: "Neither of the men were overbearing, clingy, or controlling in any way." She just didn't want to be in a romantic relationship.

Mary took seriously the disconnect between how she thought she was supposed to live her life and how she actually wanted to live. She read a lot. She went into therapy. Over time she was able to acknowledge who she really was and become comfortable with that person:

> I feel like I spent much of my twenties striving to become the person I thought society wanted me to be (white-collar job, romantic partner, vacations, apartment in a nice part of the city) and I have spent my early thirties becoming more of the person I tried to bury and hide (that adventurous, slightly rebellious, and curious girl and teen who loved to wander through the woods and do things on her own).

Flipping the Script

The expert "emphasizes that being single is perfectly reasonable and rational if that is truly what you want, but that you should never slam the door to a potential relationship shut just because you have decided that this is the lifestyle you want to lead."[84]
—*Bustle*, "How to Tell If You're Meant to Stay Single"

Though well-intended, this is the kind of advice that pressures the single at heart to doubt their love of single life and their desire to stay single. Coupled people don't get treated like that. Flip the script and you will see how unimaginable it would be for them to be offered comparable advice: The expert "emphasizes that being in a romantic relationship is perfectly reasonable and rational if that is what you truly want, but that you should never slam the door to single life just because you have decided that this is the lifestyle you want to lead."

Deliberately Pursuing Romantic Relationships That Are Likely to Fail

The stories people have told me about how they came to understand themselves as single at heart, in which they ended one relationship after another, called off engagements, and got divorced, were full of painful emotions and financial challenges to them and their partners. To me, though, they all had happy endings—people who are single at heart came to realize who they really are, and then they lived their lives authentically. But not everyone shares my enthusiasm. Some people hear these people's stories and brand them as commitment phobic.

I don't doubt that there are people who crave committed romantic relationships, yet somehow can never make them work. Some people are attracted to unavailable or unsuitable partners. When they do get the romantic relationship they so desired, they want to run away. Those people, though, are not single at heart. They really do want a serious, lasting romantic relationship. Their fear is that their relationships will fail, and they often do. That leaves them crestfallen and scared to try again.

When people who are single at heart embark upon a romantic relationship, their fear is not that it will end, but that it won't. When they choose one unavailable or unsuitable partner after another, they are not being held back by untreated psychological problems; they are, at some level, deliberately pursuing relationships destined to fail.

At three different times in his life, Daz, a thirty-eight-year-old lifelong single man from Northern England, pursued romantic relationships with women who, he thought, "would not have touched me with a hockey stick." He was wrong every time. They were all interested, and for a while, the relationships chugged along. In retrospect, Daz believes that "zoning in on unrealistic, incompatible targets was a thing of genius."

"When I look back," Daz shared, "I recognize that these were incompatible, unattainable people with whom the chances of 'success' were zero, and that was *precisely* the reason I felt the need to pursue them. These were 'safe pursuits' that were bound to end up with me where I really wanted to be, on my own."

Daz was more aware of his deliberately self-sabotaging dating strategies than most other people. Typically, people who have not yet understood themselves as single at heart start out worrying that they have a problem. They wonder whether they really are commitment phobic. It is an important distinction. People who yearn for a long-term romantic relationship but are undermined by debilitating anxiety can get psychological help. People who are single at heart need to understand that in reaching for romantic relationships, they are pursuing a goal that is not really their own. Their best life is never going to have a conventional romantic relationship at the center of it.

Once single life is more widely recognized as a meaningful, fulfilling, and enriching option, not just for the short term but for life, fewer people will feel the need to pursue romantic relationships that they don't really want. That will be good for them—and for the people who would have been their ill-fated partners.

The Pressure That Comes From Being Really Good at Romantic Relationships

Being told that we are commitment phobic is just one of the ways that the true feelings of people who are single at heart are denied or dismissed. Another is the accusation that we are just bad at romantic relationships. Maybe some of us are, especially since we are mostly uninterested in them and may have had little practice. But we are uninterested in them because we are single at heart, not because we are bad at them.

What's more, some people who are single at heart are great at romantic relationships. Andrea, a twenty-nine-year-old lifelong single woman from New York City, is one of them. She can impress not just boyfriends, but even their parents: "I fit the profile of 'girlfriend material,' so parents greet me with fascination and adoration." That has its appeal. As she shared:

> I feel driven to achieve traditional goals. For example, I was a good student. I enjoyed and cared about earning good grades and teachers' approval. Along these same lines, dating and marriage appeal to me as a project that I could approach strategically, succeed at, and be praised for. But then I remember the consequence of "winning" is (presumably) a life spent with my "catch," and my aversion to that fate is enough to spoil the appeal of the pursuit.

Single All the Way: The Pressure May Have Made Us Doubt Ourselves, But We Never Married

I wrote an essay (still have it) when I was nine years old. The theme was: 'What do I want to become when I grow up.' The summary of what I wrote: What I want is [to] travel the world and be really good at my job, I do not want to be married or have a family. Pretty much on the dot in achieving all of these—my nine-year-old self would have been so proud!
—Eva (forty-four, London, England)

For people such as Jennifer, Sophia, David, Kristin, and Mary, the process of trying out marriage or romantic coupling was illuminating. A whole different route to understanding yourself as single at heart is to settle into your single life and recognize just how comfortable and suitable a life it is. It is a path that has become more and more available over time, as people in many nations around the world are staying single longer. The age at which people first marry, if they do marry, has been creeping steadily upward. In the US, it is currently hovering around thirty for men and twenty-eight for women.[85] When it is no longer normative to be married in your early twenties, young people who are single feel less stigmatized than the single people who came before them, and less pressured to hurry up and marry. The march of time across the turn of the twenty-first century has been good to single people. In a study in which a different nationally representative sample of Germans was surveyed every six years from 1996 through 2014, each new group of people without romantic partners reported greater satisfaction with their lives than the one before.[86]

At seventy-three, Joan of Newark, Delaware, has witnessed a lot of changes in attitudes toward marriage and single life. Her understanding of her own single life has changed along with them. In a guest essay she wrote for my "Living Single" blog, she recalled the controlling and demeaning way her grandmother was treated in her marriage.[87] It was, Joan shared, "not so much a partnership as a socially sanctioned hostage situation." If that's what it meant to be married, Joan wasn't interested. In her blog post, she writes:

> Where I grew up, "Would your husband let you come to the movies on Saturday?" was a perfectly ordinary question for one woman to ask another. But in the college town where I moved after graduate school, it would have been not so much insulting as incomprehensible, as if I were speaking Latin. I got the point: marriage in my new environment was indescribably more egalitarian than what I'd known before. So . . . OK, I thought. I guess I can get married now.
>
> But time passed, and nothing was happening. Without realizing it, I was experiencing what Bella DePaulo describes as believing that you *must* want to find a partner, because supposedly everyone does: "Yet, somehow, taking specific steps to do so seems to rank somewhere between cleaning out your sock drawer and deleting old emails." Email hadn't been invented yet, but the rest was right on. Although I enjoyed the company of men, the whole go-out-there-and-look-for-a-husband thing just wasn't getting off the ground, and I didn't seem to care.
>
> All around me, well-educated, independent women were flourishing in their marriages. That made me wonder: Suppose I was missing out on something? If childhood trauma was still driving my decisions, then I wasn't really free.
>
> Clearly a job for a shrink.
>
> "If you do decide to get married," the psychologist asked one day, "what kind of man would you look for?"
>
> One with a challenging job and lots of outside interests. Does volunteer work. Plays sports. Like that.
>
> "So you'd want someone who's well-rounded and intellectually stimulating?" the therapist asked me.

No. I'd want someone who's never home.

And that was it, right there. It wasn't about financial independence or equality, which were once such a big deal for me. By then, I knew plenty of married women who had those in abundance.

But I wasn't starting with a blank slate, seeking a partner with whom to build a life. My adult identity was already established, with friends, a rewarding career, a decent income, my own home, interests that deeply engaged me—and above all, a need for privacy, solitude, and autonomy too intense for a shared life. Even the most egalitarian marriage would mean trading what I had for something else. It would change not only how I spent my days, but who I was.

Joan wanted to be who she really was. Once she understood herself as single at heart, she could live authentically. She could claim her psychologically rich, independent life as her own, unafraid that she would continue to need a psychotherapist to set her straight on that matter.

For me, understanding myself as single at heart happened in steps. Growing up, my story was like many other people's—I didn't know that wanting to be single was a thing. I looked around at all the people who were coupled or aiming for coupling and I just wasn't feeling it. For a long time I thought I was just slow. Eventually, I figured, I too would be bitten by the marriage bug. In the meantime, I tried to imagine versions of coupling that might work for me. Maybe, I thought to myself, my partner would happen to live far enough away that we could only see each other on weekends. That might be nice. We'd go out to dinner. Maybe my coupled friends who only socialized with other couples on the weekends would then include me too. I wasn't thrilled with the idea of sharing a home, even for a weekend, but it would be better than living with someone all the time.

A few years later, when I was visiting a friend at her beautiful, breezy Long Island beach house, she introduced me to the couple who turned on the next light bulb for me. The woman lived in New York. The man lived in the state of Washington, nearly three thousand miles away. They rarely saw each other. Now maybe *that* was something I could live with!

I don't know when I stopped trying to fit my life into the only script I had ever learned, the one that stuck a romantic partner at the center of it. I don't think I ever had an aha moment, when in an instant I realized that single was who I really was and I would never again consider a coupled self to be one of my possible future selves. But having lived in that psychological space for quite some time now, I can report that it is glorious.

Understanding ourselves as single at heart, regardless of the path we take to get there, is liberating. We don't need to wonder any more if there's something wrong with us or if we are going to change our minds. We can settle into the life we've loved all along, bringing our secret strengths with us and reaping the rewards that have gone unrecognized for so long.

These People Are In a Committed Romantic Relationship, But Still Identify as Single at Heart

Some people who insist that they are single at heart look like they have organized their life around a committed monogamous relationship. Some are even married. They are free from the pressures to couple up because they already are coupled. These people fall into two categories. The first is the one I expected to find: they should never have married, and they are only staying married because they believe it would be unfair to their partner to leave. The others, however, love their partner and want to stay in their relationship, but still feel that, at heart, they are single. They typically don't score as high on the quiz as the single at heart people who do not have an important romantic partner in their life.

The people who are in a serious coupled relationship and stay in that relationship reluctantly sometimes tell me that they love their romantic partner and their romantic partner loves them, yet they yearn to be single. One man said he thought it would sound "crazy" to suggest that a person could be in a loving and respectful marriage but still feel that their "authentic self is calling them" to single life; but that was exactly how he felt. Looking back at when he was single, he saw that as a more expansive life, one that validated his values and fostered his strengths. For example, he deeply valued the loving friendships he had nurtured when he was single, but as a married man he felt that "they needed to be secondary in the hierarchy of my affection, and that has its effects on intimacy and growth." He stayed married but he felt that he was resigning himself "to a satisfactory life, leaving the extraordinary life by the wayside."

Eleanore, a sixty-four-year-old from Sydney, Australia, tells a very different story. She is in a "lovely romantic relationship" with a man and wants to stay in that relationship. The two of them don't live together, but they have been a couple for years. Eleanore is an introvert and in social situations, she appreciates having a partner who will "go with me to help take the edge off or save me from having to interact with others when I don't really want to." She also likes sex and "having someone to travel with, fix things, kill bugs."

Having a place of her own is important to Eleanore. "I enjoy my own company and like spending time alone. I love that my time and my money are my own and I can spend them however I want without having to consult with anyone. (Choosing to do so sometimes is different versus having to or being expected to.)"

"Early in my current relationship," Eleanore said, "my guy expressed a desire to see more of me. I asked, 'How much more?' and he responded that he wouldn't mind seeing me every day. I thought to myself, *Why in the world would anyone want to see someone every day?* until it dawned on me that this is what so many people in the world want. I've never wanted that."

"I've always valued my singledom over being part of a couple," she added. "It's a bit of a juggling act."

In her commitment to having time and space to herself, Eleanore is 100 percent single at heart. She demonstrates this by choosing to live apart from her partner. Every person I heard from who identified as single at heart even though they had a significant romantic partner either lived in a place of their own, in separate sections of a house, shared a home only until they could afford a place of their own, or spent long periods of time apart.

Eleanore also enjoys the independence of having her own money and spending it as she wishes, without consulting with her partner or anyone else. That is characteristic of people who are single at heart.

One of the quiz questions was, "When you are thinking about making a big change in your life, such as embarking on a new career or moving across the country, which do you prefer?" Eleanore rejected the answer "Making the decision with a partner, even if that means that you do not pursue your favorite option." She instead chose "Making the decision that feels right to you, without worrying about whether a partner would approve, or whether your decision might stand in the way of a partner's goals." Next to that, she wrote, "This is my 'real' response, though it may not be fair to my partner, and I *possibly* would take his needs into consideration." That's the ambivalence of someone who identifies as single at heart and yet values her romantic partner and does not want to be unfair to him.

In some ways, Eleanore sees herself as having the best of both worlds. In response to the question of whether she is self-sufficient, meaning that she likes handling problems and challenges mostly on her own, she said yes. Then she added, "but I'm not above letting him take over things I don't want to do." Another quiz question asked, "Think about the possibility that when you go to sleep at night, there might not be anyone else in bed with you. How does that make you feel?" She chose both options: "You would not like that" *and* "You are fine with that." She explained: "I like sleeping alone. It can also be emotionally comforting having him there sometimes. Because we live separately, I get both."

Our Role Models

When I was around nine or ten years old, I was impressed with my town's Girls' Club director, June Bowman. She had an office, carried a briefcase, had her own car, and was the boss. Back then, she was my idol. When I was a kid, I wanted to be June Bowman.

—Claudia (sixty-nine, Washington, DC)

Protections from the Pressures

Claudia had what many single people only wish they had: a role model. She knew it was possible to live an exciting life as a single person because she knew someone who already did, someone she idolized. Role models, supportive teachers and friends, communities of like-minded members, astute therapists, and enlightened talks, writings, and podcasts can all provide protections from the relentless pressures to put a romantic partner at the center of our lives.

Ketaki (thirty-four, Manipal, India) grew up amid thousands of role models. Most of her teachers were lifelong single people who were devoted to their students and passionate about teaching. They were part of a spiritual community in South India that discouraged marriage. When I hear from single people in the United States who are religious, I know just what to expect. They are pained by the ways their religious communities seem to value and validate married people more than single people. The lifelong single people who were Ketaki's role models, though, believed that "a diversity of ways of living and child-rearing was necessary for human progress." From them, Ketaki was "able to draw on a rich legacy of single life."[88]

In most places around the world, communities of single people who support and validate other single people are rare. We single people may need to create our own special spaces. In the Community of Single People

Facebook group, we share our joys and our accomplishments, discuss the kinds of issues particularly relevant to single life, and unreservedly express our exasperation at the ways in which single people are stereotyped, stigmatized, pitied, or ignored.[89]

In a discussion of what the group has meant to many of the members, Selene said:

> I was a serial dater and buying into the myth that I had to find "the one" (while not really feeling that in my heart of hearts). I suddenly found this entire world where the whole cultural narrative of romance and marriage was no longer important but living an authentic life was. The conversations and perspectives in this group have been invaluable to me. I love both feeling that I've found kindred souls *and* the spirited debates where we don't always agree.

Single people sometimes look to therapists for support for staying single. That doesn't always work because some therapists assume that their single clients would be mentally healthier if they became coupled, even when those clients do not describe their single status as a problem. But the best mental health professionals can be magnificently insightful.

In *The Art of Not Falling Apart*, Christina Patterson did not try to hide the deep yearning to be coupled that she experienced for years, or her many attempts to unsingle herself. Her therapist wasn't buying it:

> "I don't think," said the shrink one day, "that you actually want to meet someone." . . . I was shocked. What do you *mean* I don't want to meet someone? What about all the dating? The bloody awful dating? What about the speed dating, and the internet dating, and the dating agency, and the blind dates arranged by friends, and the dinners, and the parties, and all that sheer, exhausting, humiliating effort? . . . But the

more I thought about it, the more I realized he was probably right. The fact is that I often ran away because I was bored. When I'm on my own, I'm never, ever bored.[90]

The people who know us best can be among the most supportive, once they realize that single life really is our best life. Evan (forty, San Francisco, California) like many others, described experiencing less pressure and more validation as he grew older:

> Especially when I was younger, people used to say patronizing things like, "Oh you'll change your mind" or "You just haven't met the right guy yet." As I've gotten older, though, I've heard these comments less often. I think the people around me have realized this is who I really am.

We can also be selective about who we welcome into our inner circles. As Sonya, age forty-seven, of Parkersburg, West Virginia, said, "The great thing about being single is I can choose my people, and choose who to avoid."

Being Single at Heart: Is It Hardwired?

I can't provide a definitive answer to the question of whether being single at heart is hardwired. More research is needed. But I can say that the single at heart life is more than just a lifestyle. It is deeper than that. People who are unambivalently single at heart are powerfully drawn to single life; for them, that is the life that feels most natural, comfortable, and authentic. I often focus on the people who identify most definitively as single at heart, but I see the single at heart status as existing on a spectrum. Some people are more clearly single at heart than others.

Someone who is not single at heart but wants to be cannot simply will themselves into that way of being. However, anyone can try out the single at heart life. For example, they can try to appreciate solitude and make the most of whatever freedom they may have. They can attend fondly to all the people who matter to them, rather than just prioritizing a romantic partner. Occasionally, that experiment can be revelatory, as when people come to realize that single life really is their best life.

Advice

What can we do to create a more welcoming world for the single at heart, so we feel supported in embracing our best single life rather than pressured to unsingle ourselves? Here is some advice, first, for our allies, who want the best for us but may be unsure how to make that happen; second, for people who are intrigued by single life but have concerns; and third, for my single at heart soulmates.

For Our Allies

Ask about something other than romantic relationships.
Have you just been introduced to someone? Where are they from? Have they lived here long? How do they know the hosts? That was quite the storm yesterday, wasn't it? With so many potential conversational gambits, there is no need to alight on marital or relationship status. People who want you to know that they have a spouse or romantic partner will work that into the conversation, whether you are interested or not.

The experience of Sophia, (fifty-seven, England) shows what it could mean to someone who is single at heart not to be asked that predictable question:

> I was divorced at forty-three. When I was forty-six, I attended
> a friend's birthday party. I met a woman and I chatted with
> her for about fifteen minutes. At some point in the conver-
> sation a light bulb went on . . . she had not inquired about
> my relationship status! I realized that I was actually cringing
> inside waiting for her to ask me if I was dating anyone. It

was remarkable that she had not tried to determine whether I was partnered! So I said to her, "Thank you for not asking whether or not I'm in a relationship. Somehow that makes me feel really great." And she said very matter-of-factly, "You are a whole person unto yourself." And I almost cried because of the truth of it.

Don't ask single people why they are still single.
When people ask why we are still single, it can seem like harmless small talk. But this question can be infuriating, offensive, and sometimes devastating. Laurie, age thirty-five, of Michigan, told this story:

> Sometimes people come right out and ask if I'm seeing anyone, while others might ask, "What's new?" if they haven't seen me in a while, but you can tell what they're really wondering about is my love life. I once had a doctor question me about why I wasn't married. "What's going on? You're pretty. You shouldn't have any trouble. Do people think you're weird?" (He actually said that.) And it continued. So many assumptions: That I wanted to be in a relationship/get married, that my life would somehow be better if I was, that something must be wrong with me socially that I wasn't married by a certain age. That was a big slap in the face that pushed me to date and probably kept me in the dating pool when I didn't want to be there.

I've written some popular blog posts compiling single people's favorite answers to the "why are you single" question. Witty retorts such as "just lucky, I guess" and "I'm overqualified" can be satisfying. But they can be dismissed as jokes, or worse, interpreted as defensive. I have a fondness for a nonconfrontational, "just curious" sort of approach that gently, casually asks the other person to rethink their most fundamental assumptions. I like the suggestion offered by Kris Marsh, author of *The Love Jones Cohort: Single and Living Alone in the Black Middle Class*: ask the person, "What do you mean by that?"[91] The person faced with that question soon realizes that it is difficult to justify the "why are you single" question.

Be happy for us.
The single at heart are not disconsolate when our friends or relatives find the partner of their dreams (unless, of course, they go on to erase us from their lives). We are not secretly envious of them. We don't want to steal their spouse. We are happy to be happy for them and wish they would understand us and be happy for us. That, it turns out, can be a lot to ask. Here's what Joan (seventy-three, Newark, Delaware) said:

> A few years ago I introduced two widowed professors to each other and they subsequently got married. A few of our mutual colleagues commiserated with me on missing out, as if I'd been left at the gate while the other woman got the guy. *That is an aspect of living single that I could easily do without.* No matter how often I say it, even people who've known me for a long time can't get their minds around the reality that I really, really want to live as I do. What I wish I had from the world of committed romantic relationships is universal recognition of the validity of my way of life.

Understand that we are not just marking time.
Sometimes people have no trouble believing that single people genuinely want to be single *for a while*. Especially when they are young. Or while they are getting over a divorce or breakup. But that desire to be single is presumed to be temporary. It shouldn't be. Here's what some coupled coworkers said to Andrea (twenty-nine, New York City):

People at Club Med would always say, "What a cool life! You're smart to do this while you can!" as if someone is coming for me to force me to settle down. Do these people realize the life path that they've chosen (and regret?) is optional?

Let children be children.
Don't ask five-year-olds if they have a boyfriend or girlfriend. Fathers, don't tell your daughters you want to live long enough to walk them down the aisle. Parents and relatives, be attuned to and validate who your children really are and what they really want, and continue to do so even when they are grown. Speak to children about the choices they have in adult life, and give single life the same attention and respect as other life paths.

Feature the single at heart in your creative work.
If you are a member of the creative class, write novels, movies, TV shows, and song lyrics that feature themes other than marriage plots and romance. Show us complex, fascinating people who are single at heart. Reveal what they are really thinking when cast among the masses still unabashedly squealing at the latest engagement announcement. You will have the next comedic hit!

For People Who Are Intrigued by Single Life, But Have Concerns

Try it, you might like it.
Just about all the life stories I have shared in this chapter ended the same way: the protagonists realized that despite all the pressures to couple up, single life is their best life, and they then live accordingly. Maybe you have read all those stories, feel intrigued by them, but still feel uncertain as to whether single life would be your most meaningful and fulfilling life. The best way to know for sure is to try it. Commit to living single, perhaps for a year. When the time is up, you will know.

It's your life; what you want matters most.

Some people, such as "Happy Singleness," the person who wrote to advice columnist Carolyn Hax, already know that they love being single. Her problem is that her grown kids are urging her to unsingle herself and the pressures to do so seem to be ubiquitous. People like "Happy Singleness" deserve to take control of their lives. They know themselves best. They should honor the person they know themselves to be.

For the Single at Heart

Live your single life fully and joyfully.

To get to the point where you understand that single life is your best life and then identify as single at heart, you have overcome a whole system of rewards and punishments and norms, expectations, and ideologies that tried to persuade you that only coupled life is normal, natural, and truly fulfilling. Now do everything you always wanted to do as a single person. Take your rightful place in society. There is nothing you should hesitate to do just because you are single.

Own your love of single life.

On *The Drew Barrymore Show*, Barrymore had a question for the actress Allison Janney, then sixty-one: "You have put out there in the world that you are not looking to get married or have children—is this the truth?" "Yeah," Janney replied. "I think if I would have found the right guy at the right time who wanted to have kids, I probably would have with the right partner, 'cause I wasn't ever really confident that I wanted to have kids. I would rather regret not having kids than have kids and regret that. I really am at this time in my life getting to know who I am and what I want. I'd love to find—eventually find—someone to share my life with, but if it doesn't happen, I'll be just fine. But it would be nice."[92]

Whenever I hear comments like Janney gave, I wonder about the hedging. Is it possible that she really wanted to leave it at, "Yes, it is true that I'm not looking to get married or have children."? Did she feel that, even with all the freedom that her celebrity status granted her, it wouldn't be acceptable to give such a blunt answer without qualifications?

Maybe it really is true for Allison Janney that she would have married and had kids if the right person had come along at the right time, and that she would still love to find a life partner. But those of us who have been single all our lives are expected to justify our lives and we know it. If Janney's life had unfolded differently, Barrymore would likely not have asked her the analogous question: "You have put out there in the world that you are not looking to leave your marriage or stop being involved in the lives of your children—is this the truth?"

I also wonder about the hedging because people who really are not looking to marry or have kids have told me that they've done the same thing. They can only go so far in admitting how they really feel. Mary (thirty-three, Buffalo, New York) told me this story:

> I was eating lunch with a coworker who I didn't know very well on a personal level. Our conversation turned to the topic of marriage, and I remember feeling comfortable telling her that I didn't see the point of marriage, that I thought it was an outdated institution used to privilege some people, etc. When she asked me if I would like to at least have a committed long-term romantic partner in my life even if we did not marry, I said, "Oh yes, of course!" even though I knew I was lying. I felt like there was no way that I could admit that I was completely content to be single forever, because it made me seem like a freak. Being ideologically at odds with the tradition of marriage was one thing, but rejecting the entire lifelong monogamous partner paradigm seemed way too radical a thing to confess.

Mary's concerns were warranted. When Kristin (fifty-five, Bellingham, Washington) decided that she was going to tell her friends and family that she was single at heart, she wasn't worried, but she should have been:

> I hadn't thought I needed any preparation for that announcement. I didn't imagine for a minute that I would be ostracized! The lesbian community moved away from me like I had a communicable disease. If I wasn't "on the market," what was the point? My family was oddly reticent about the announcement. It didn't make sense to them. People are supposed to pair up, and they didn't care who I paired up with, but to make a conscious choice *not* to pair up was just weird. Friends asked incredibly rude and personal questions, like did that mean I'm asexual? They felt entitled to ask questions about my sexuality when for me to ask them similar questions would be unthinkable. ("How often do you and Fred have sex? Do you ever wish you were with someone else?") And of course, they wanted to figure out what was "wrong" and "fix me." It is easier for most people to accept the notion of a same-sex couple than the notion of not being in a couple at all. It gives them some satisfaction to accept you as a gay person, they get some liberal validation from it. Single at heart gives them nothing but a good long scary look at their own situation.

Both Mary and Kristin may have been treated more warmly if they said they felt sorry for themselves for being single. I'm grateful to Mary for taking the first step of telling her colleague that she was uninterested in marriage. Maybe at some point she will be ready to go all the way and say that she is also uninterested in having a long-term romantic partner in her life. I'm proud of Kristin for declaring herself single at heart. She didn't get the reaction either of us would have liked, but I bet she made an impression, and maybe sharing her story will help change the reception for those who come after her. Her mother and her friends, perhaps for the first time, had to take seriously the idea that some single people love being single and are not looking to change that. Now they know someone for whom that is true; it isn't just an abstraction.

It is on us, the single at heart, to own our singlehood. When we answer questions about our single lives straightforwardly, without qualification or apology, we normalize living single. When we effuse about our passions, or the people who mean so much to us, or wax poetic about savoring solitude, we model a joyful and celebratory way of being single.

There are also rewards for us when we own our love of being single. Here's how Joan (seventy-three, Newark, Delaware) described her experiences:

> As a professor in a big public university, I encountered less singlism than I might have, but heaven knows it was still there. For years, I sorted out each separate issue—like having trouble getting a credit card and later a mortgage—and then forgot about it. Without fully realizing it, I tended not to make an issue of being single, as if not wanting to get the marrieds started. The less said, the better, it seemed. But a few years ago, when I started writing about being single, I felt whole for the first time. It's not entirely comparable to a homosexual coming out of the closet, since everyone knew all along that I was single. But I felt the same sense of liberation and self-affirmation that I've heard gays and lesbians express about taking one's full, rightful place without diffidence or apology—in my case, as a heterosexual woman who prefers to live single and is damn good at it.

When I meet new people, I make it a point to describe myself as a lifelong single person. At a housewarming party in my neighborhood, when a married man introduced himself to me, I replied, "I'm Bella, I'm sixty-nine, and I have been single my whole life." I meant it as a statement of pride. But in response, he told me about a woman who had been contentedly single her whole life, then got married at sixty-five and has been living happily ever since. I think he was trying to reassure me, as if to say, "Don't worry, Bella. Even in your sixties, you could still find The One." I told him I prefer stories in which the happy single people stay single, then added that I thought marriage was overrated. He thought for a moment, gazed at his wife who was out of earshot, and said, "If I admitted how I felt about that, I'd spend the night in the shed."

3

Freedom

I am in a wonderful place in my life. Single for fifteen years now, and
counting every second as a deep, personal blessing not to be squandered.
When I was in Sydney and my relationship ended, I had to suddenly learn
to do all of those things that someone else had taken care of.
I found a new home, moved house, and learned to drive.
I taught myself how to write HTML and created a website for a rock
band in the UK. The band members and I shared a passion for music,
and I took a trip to the UK and met them. There I found a social life,
overcoming a deep discomfort with socializing and discovering an ability
to connect not only to other people, but to bring other people together. I
gave up my career in Australia and moved to the UK to be
closer to the music I love and those who make it. I met more and more
musicians (they used to be just names on the backs of my records and
CDs), brought them together to play, organized their gigs and venues,
photographed and video recorded them, have had my photography
featured on CDs, etc. . . . And now, quite suddenly and unexpectedly, to
my utter delight, I am actually playing onstage with these musicians.
I have become a rock chick at the age of fifty-one!
—Carol (London, England)

All her life Carol felt called to the freedom and autonomy of single
life. Even as a child, she told me, she "instinctively knew" that she
did not want to be coupled. But for the longest time, she never questioned
the presumption that coupling is what everyone did. Dutifully she did it

too, even moving in with a man. It didn't work. The whole time, she felt "markedly detached" from her partner and from coupled life. When she was thirty-six, the two of them parted amicably, and that's when her real single at heart life began.

Carol embraced her single life wholeheartedly. She learned new skills, including practical life skills and skills she could monetize. She honed her gift for photography and got to see her work featured on the backs of CDs. She discovered a talent for socializing and for bringing people together that she never knew she had. She followed her passion for music, all the way from one continent to another. Her story wasn't of a lovesick fan besotted by some cool musician dude. Her love was for the music, and *she* became the cool rock chick, up onstage in London, having the time of her life.

For Carol, coupled life was a smaller life. Once she was free of it, she went from being a reticent person who did not know how to drive to a performing musician whose life became "a delightful whirl of busyness." Embracing single life liberated Carol from the expectation that her adult life would follow a predetermined script of moving in with a romantic partner and getting married, having kids and grandkids. She was free to write her own script for how her adult life would unfold, and if, at any point, she wanted to rewrite it, she could do that too.

After my father died, I got a sympathy card that included a handwritten note from a woman who shared that when her father died, her mother blossomed. I thought it was an odd way to express sympathy. Then a few days later, I got another note that expressed the same thing. I still didn't understand it. Now I think I do. Some women (and men) live their biggest, fullest, most authentic, and most meaningful lives when they are single. Alongside the profound grief that many widowed people experience is something else: the sense that a new life is about to begin, one in which they may well flourish.

It is different for newly single people who yearn to be coupled. They rarely do what Carol did. They instead prioritize finding that one special person. Even those single people who want to be coupled but don't feel desperate about it, and who promise themselves that they will make the best of the time they spend single, don't invest in their single lives as fully, joyfully, and unreservedly as Carol did.

In theory single people who want to be coupled have freedom too. In theory coupled people with supportive partners can pursue their dreams and maybe even get some encouragement and financial backstopping along the way. And some really do. But freedom typically does not have the same place in their lives that it does for the single at heart.

I asked the forty-one people who shared their life stories with me a simple question, "What do you like best about living single?" It was an open-ended question; in response, they could have said anything at all. Every one of them, in some way or another, highlighted the same thing: freedom.

In a survey of more than two hundred thousand adults from thirty-one European countries, many people, both married and unmarried, said that freedom was important to them, as were other individualistic values such as creativity and trying new things.[93] Valuing freedom paid emotional dividends: The people who cared more about values such as freedom and creativity were happier. Tellingly, the people who were not married cared about values such as freedom even more than the married people did. And they got even more happiness out of their embrace of freedom. The link between valuing freedom and feeling happy was stronger for them.

The single at heart get more out of their freedom because they do more with it. They take advantage of the opportunities their freedom offers them to learn and to grow, to care for the people who mean the most to them, to contribute to their communities and make a difference, to choose meaningful work, and to be the captains of their own life ships.

Learning and Growing

> As a single guy, you are in a much better position to think, ponder, seek
> deeper understanding, question things, learn, and grow (intellectually,
> spiritually, philosophically, etc.). Personally, this is a big one for me,
> and it's something I wouldn't live without.[94]
> —Ed Anderson, *Good Bachelorhood blog*

Most nights, I stay up until 4 a.m., sometimes later. That's been true my entire adult life. Those long stretches of time, when it is dark out, my friends are asleep, and no one is expecting me to return an email or a text, are when I do some of my best thinking and writing. At night, my life becomes a life of the mind, and like Ed, I wouldn't have it any other way.

For some who are single at heart, our love of learning can be focused, intense, and motivating. Sonya (forty-seven, Parkersburg, West Virginia) said, "Once I have an idea, I must see it through to the end—often until the wee hours of the morning."

Ginny, age fifty-nine, of Ontario, Canada, loves the natural world, and has aimed her rapt attention on one element of that world after another. "I love learning and am currently focused on moths," she shared. "Over the last month, I've been outside at the moth light every month, taking over three thousand photos of moths."

On the single at heart quiz, the single at heart are more likely to say that they have a sense of personal mastery (a can-do attitude) and that they are self-sufficient (they like handling problems and challenges mostly on their own). Sonya, for example, is a DIY goddess, who shared, "Because I live alone I have acquired an arsenal of diverse skills. I can handle basic carpentry, electrical and plumbing repair, cooking, sewing, landscaping, and financial planning." Those kinds of competencies are among our secret strengths. Because we have learned to do so many of these things, or figured out ways of getting them done, we are often thriving in our old age, when some other people, such as the newly widowed or newly divorced, are struggling to learn some of those skills for the first time.

If you were to track the emotions of single and married people, you would find that in both groups, people with a greater sense of personal mastery are less likely to report negative feelings. Lifelong single people, though, benefit more: they get even more protection from feeling down if they have more of a can-do attitude, research shows. The groups diverge even more in what they get out of their self-sufficiency. For lifelong single people, the more they like handling challenges mostly on their own, the less likely they are to experience negative emotions. For longtime married people, though, the reverse is true. The more self-sufficient they are, the more likely they are to feel down.[95]

> If you travel with another person, it is the relationship that is put to the test. If you go by yourself, it is the relationship with yourself that is put to the test, and there is where growth happens.
>
> —Eva (forty-four, London, England)

Eva thinks of herself as "an adventurer, explorer, unconventional life-lover." She cares deeply about climate justice, women's rights, and animal rights and she loves art, nature, design, and food. When she was thirty-four and living in London, though, she was burned out at work and her creativity was flagging. She wasn't living up to the person she wanted to be, and she wanted to do something about that. Something big, the sort of thing most people only dream of. She wanted to take an entire year to travel the world; in her words, "to lose myself to find my path again."

After a year of preparation, off she went, first to South Africa, Zimbabwe, and Namibia, then India, then China. Vietnam, Cambodia, and Thailand were next, followed by Australia and New Zealand, and finally Costa Rica. All along the way, she honored the values she long held dear, and rediscovered her passions. She did volunteer work with rescued elephants and horses, worked with children to raise awareness about environmental issues, and volunteered at a conservation center. She taught courses on English as a foreign language and took courses on women's issues, language, culture, calligraphy, and cooking. She explored villages and cities and made friends on every continent she visited—friends who, to this day, are still a part of her life.

Eva didn't have a ton of money, so for the year before the trip, she bought almost nothing and rarely went out. Then during her travels, she shared rooms and tried a lot of inexpensive street food. She had prepared herself physically too in that year leading up to her travels, working on her strength and her fitness. She read voraciously and planned carefully.

An item on the single at heart quiz asked, "When you are thinking about making a big change in your life, such as embarking on a new career or moving across the country, which do you prefer?" Nearly everyone who was clearly single at heart, 96 percent, chose "Making the decision that feels right to you, without worrying about whether a partner would approve, or whether your decision might stand in the way of a partner's goals." In contrast, 70 percent who were not single at heart said they preferred "making the decision with a partner, even if that means that you do not get to pursue your favorite option."

For Eva, making the decision on her own and then planning and traveling on her own were key to the joyfulness, psychological richness, and authenticity of that magical year. "It was the extended alone time that allowed me to think, reflect, observe and recharge," she said. When, as a woman traveling alone, she faced down many challenges and survived some harrowing experiences, she was rewarded with "an immense sense of empowerment every time I was able to say, 'I did it!'"

Freedom, Eva knows, "is not just doing what you want." It was also, for her, an opportunity to learn a tremendous amount about other people, other places, and other ways of thinking—a hallmark of a psychologically rich life. "I also learned how to create happiness for myself and to own my happiness," she added, "and this is the essence of freedom."

Our Role Models

Gracious was my teacher from age twelve to seventeen. In addition to teaching piano, she owned a jazz club in our town and each year would host our recitals there. She had a bunch of rescue animals that wandered around her house during my lessons and didn't have any children. She was definitely an anomaly among the women in my world. Almost all of the women I knew were married, had been married, or were on their way to marriage. I was intrigued by Gracious's life: she lived alone, had her own business, and looked to be doing exactly what she wanted to do. She moved to France around the same time I went off to college, and I was struck by her willingness to uproot her life and move somewhere new in middle age. To me, she lived a life that was liberating and fulfilling and, after having found my own way to singleness, I often think that she, unknowingly, was a positive influence and model for me. She showed me what a single life could be.

—Elizabeth (forty-seven, Newport, Rhode Island)

Charting Our Own Life Courses

In 1953, the year I was born, the psychologist Robert Havighurst published his influential model of the stages of adult life. He proclaimed that the tasks of early adulthood were selecting a mate, learning to live with a spouse, and starting a family.[96] That way of thinking erased people like me who never selected a mate, never had to learn to live with a spouse, and never started a family (at least not in the conventional sense). It probably contributed to the stereotyping of single people as not fully adult.

Other stage models were proposed after that, and then, in academic circles, they fell out of favor. Northwestern University professor Dan McAdams, one of the leading scholars of adult development and identity, told me that "the big problem is that stage theories do not accommodate nonnormative life paths. And as it turns out, nonnormative life paths are more and more the norm."

Outside of academia, the old-fashioned stage model from the 1950s still guides many people's expectations about how adult life should unfold. Some like the structure it provides. They appreciate having a clear path to follow.

Not the single at heart. We love the freedom of setting aside conventions and charting our own life path. The stages of our lives can include traveling the world (as Eva did), moving to another country in midlife (as Gracious did), or following some other path that is uniquely our own. For instance, when I asked Sonya (forty-seven, Parkersburg, West Virginia) how she would describe the stages of her life, she said:

> Mine has gone something like this: bachelor's degree; establish career; side hustles; author/artist/designer; godmother; master's degree; National Board Certification; homeowner; assuming leadership roles in union and community organizations; godmother duties waning as kids grow up; maintain career; caring for older people; more focus on personal health and interests; retirement planning; travel; whatever I damn well please!

There is no one sequence of life stages for people who are single. Within the constraints of our resources and opportunities, the possibilities are limitless, and those of us who are single at heart find that liberating and exciting.

Flipping the Script

"I've been completely single for over eleven years with only one
relationship before then. About three years ago I started solo traveling
for the first time, and there I discovered an intense joy I felt while being
completely alone. I believe it was actually life changing.
However, sometimes the longing for love, for romantic connection,
still comes up. And occasionally it gets so strong that sometimes
I wonder if all the traveling, all the fun things I do by myself, are really
just a way to fill the hole in my life when what I actually want is a
relationship. How do we know if we really like being single or if
we're just covering up a void of not having a relationship?"

—Simon

I told Simon, "I don't think there is an obvious answer to your question, but I
do think that cultural conditioning makes it way more likely that we will think
we crave romantic relationships than to think we crave solitude."

Imagine if we flipped the script, and Simon instead asked this: "About
three years ago, I got married for the first time and discovered an intense joy
I felt from my connection to my spouse. I believe it was actually life changing.
However, sometimes my longing for what I had when I was single still comes up.
And occasionally it gets so strong that sometimes I wonder if all the attention I
am lavishing on my spouse, and all that I invest in my marriage, are just a way
to fill the hole in my life when what I actually want is to be single."

Until Simon's question and my flipped version of it are equally
plausible, people who love their single lives are going to feel more pressure to
doubt themselves than people who love being coupled will. And that means
that neither single people nor coupled people are totally free to know what
they really want and to live their most authentic lives.

Doing Meaningful Work

I am mostly retired now, managing my own small business taking care of animals. It has been my favorite way to earn money ever. When I told people I was leaving corporate to have a pet sitting business, *no one* was impressed, or even happy for me. They thought if I hired others, then I would be a manager again, and that would be impressive. I told them if I did that, I would just be managing people with all that stress, which I hated, and they would get to spend all the time with the animals.

—Peggy (sixty-seven, Atlanta, Georgia)

Despite all the cultural messaging insisting that it is marriage and romantic coupling that is most essential to have a life that is fulfilling, most adults in the US disagree. When asked in a 2019 Pew Research Center survey whether each of a number of factors was essential to live a fulfilling life, only 16 percent of men and 17 percent of women said that marriage was essential, and just 26 percent of men and 30 percent of women said that being in a committed relationship was essential. The one factor endorsed far more often than any other was having a job or career that you enjoy. Fifty-seven percent of men and 46 percent of women said that was essential.[97]

Enjoyable work, or meaningful work, may not always be the most lucrative work. I think it would be totally understandable if single people cared about money more than coupled people do, especially if they live alone and have to cover all expenses on their own. In a striking analysis published in *The Atlantic*, Lisa Arnold and Christina Campbell estimated that a single woman, compared to a married woman, can incur more than a million dollars in extra costs over the course of her adult life. Those penalties in housing costs, health care costs, taxation, and Social Security—which are not specific to women—are written right into the laws of the US government and the policies of private companies.[98]

And yet study after study has shown that single people prioritize meaning over materialism. For example, when more than fifteen thousand

Americans were asked to rank a list of job features, married people were especially likely to put income high on their list. Single people were more likely to prioritize other things, such as having work that "is important and gives a feeling of accomplishment."[99]

In a study of more than seven hundred Midwesterners in their late twenties, the people who had been single their whole lives, more so than those who had married, said that they valued meaningful work. The married people cared more about money, job security, and opportunities for advancement.[100]

What made that study remarkable is that the same people were asked the same questions about what mattered to them back when they were in high school and no one was married. Even then, the people who would stay single at least until their late twenties were already saying that they cared about having work that was meaningful, while the people who would go on to marry already valued money and job security more.

An item on the single at heart quiz asked, "If you had to choose between meaningful work that did not pay much or uninspiring work that paid a lot, which would you pick?" Of the people who were clearly single at heart, 76 percent chose meaningful work. Of course, we do have to support ourselves. David (sixty-five, Austin, Texas) said, "I might work the big money for a while, then turn back to the meaningful."

And for some of us, it can take a while to deprogram ourselves from more conventional ways of thinking. As Donna, a forty-nine-year-old resident of Seattle, Washington, explained, "I used to think I needed to constantly make more money, to get promotions and raises, and attain more. And then I asked myself why am I doing this? Is it because I want it or because I'm supposed to want it? I realize now that I have everything I want and more than I need."

As soon as Ginny (fifty-nine, Ontario, Canada) completed her graduate education, she found work befitting her superb credentials. She was hired by a department of microbiology and immunology, then worked for the federal government under the North American Free Trade Agreement, registering pesticides in the US, Mexico, and twenty other countries. The work paid her bills but did not feed her soul. She quit and never looked back. Soon she staked out a place at a farmers' market, contentedly selling her homemade jams, jellies, and chutneys, as well as cards and artwork featuring her photography. When her mother developed dementia, Ginny relocated to be closer to her. There she found "the greatest job" of all for someone like her, who has always been enthralled by the natural world. She conducts bird surveys for a local land trust. "I get paid to watch birds while standing in a pasture in excellent weather," she shared.

Work can be meaningful when it makes a difference. MaryL, a sixty-two-year-old from Los Angeles, California, told me, "I was very fortunate to have figured out early in my work career that I needed to know that I was contributing to being a part of the solution instead of the problem. I stopped chasing the purse (money), then I looked forward to getting up every day and going to work." Acadia (thirty-six, Melbourne, Australia) said, "I am a public servant and I love that I can, in a very small way, make my country a better place."

Just as single people get more happiness out of their embrace of freedom than married people do, and more protection from negative feelings out of their sense of personal mastery and self-sufficiency, so too do they get more satisfaction out of work that is fulfilling and meaningful, and from their feelings of accomplishment. In the survey of hundreds of thousands of adults from thirty-one European nations, the lifelong single people were especially likely to enjoy a happiness dividend from work that was deeply satisfying.[101] Meaningful work can be a boon to anyone's fulfillment, but lifelong single people seem to benefit the most.

Financial Freedom

I love that my time and my money are my own and I can spend them however I want without having to consult with anyone.

—Eleanore (sixty-four, Sydney, Australia)

Asked what advice she would give to young people, the award-winning novelist Sandra Cisneros said she would tell them to earn their own money. "You can't follow your dream if someone else is giving you your money," she said.[102] People who are single at heart get to choose meaningful work over lucrative work because they have their own money and the financial freedom that comes with it. Decisions about money are their own. Mary (thirty-three, Buffalo, New York) said, "I would not have been able to quit my human services job last year as easily as I did. I think if I was married I would have another person's finances to consider."

Single people also have the freedom to pursue opportunities that require financial resources if that's what they prefer. In "Unmarried and Unbothered," Keturah Kendrick profiled black women who valued freedom more than marriage. Of one of the women she interviewed, a sixty-two-year-old lifelong single woman with no children, Kendrick said, "She has been able to take career risks, stockpile savings, make use of expendable income, and invest in her own business." She did have romantic relationships when she was younger, but "none of those relationships meant more to [her] than the freedom to control her own finances, career trajectory, and overall movements throughout life."[103]

The financial freedom of single life is also a freedom from the risks of building a life with a less economically adept romantic partner. When Julie, a forty-four-year-old from Raleigh, North Carolina, was in her thirties, she felt a lot of pressure to date. Her longest relationship was with an older man who she described as a good person who never tried to control her. However, he was broke and in debt. He had no savings, no retirement money, and he did not make a lot of money at his job. He proposed, but they never married. Julie explained, "I worked two jobs, saved up for retirement, worked overtime until my hands hurt, and made wise investments long before we met." They split, and Julie has never had any regrets. She realized she appreciates being single and can stay that way. When asked what she now likes best about single life, she had a long list; the first item was, "Making financial decisions on my own and not having to explain those decisions to anyone."

Becoming the Deciders

I love deciding everything about my life.
—Amy (forty-four, Frisco, Texas)

The single at heart love being the deciders. In our work lives, for example, many of us want to do our work in our own time and in our own ways. It helps to be our own bosses or to have the kind of job where we don't get bossed around all that much. Joan, the seventy-three-year-old retired professor in Newark, Delaware, said, "A very important element of my work life is that I had a great deal of autonomy. As long as I got the job done—publications, teaching, student evals, creating new courses, committees—nobody cared when I did it, or where, or what I was wearing at the time. Also important was the opportunity to reinvent myself to follow new interests."

Jennifer (forty-five, Denver, Colorado) has worked in the corporate world and could have managed people, but chose to work mostly on her own. She has also pursued self-employment, where she has the freedom to do her work wherever she likes, which is often remotely.

Steve, a thirty-nine-year-old from Bolton, England, is an indefatigable adventurer who has run marathons and half-marathons in fourteen countries, including Norway, host of the most northerly half-marathon in the world, and probably the coldest. Steve used to work in an office, but found that stressful and dispiriting. "Now, as a translator, I've become my own boss and I don't employ anyone." Steve has to work longer hours to support himself than he did in his previous job, but it is worth it. He treasures the opportunity to work at his own pace and when he wants to head to some far-flung outpost, he can take his work with him. "I find the adage is true—find a job you enjoy, and you don't really work. For me, it is playing with words. I get paid to play with words. I'm a very lucky man nowadays."

In his analyses of the survey data from thirty-one European nations, sociologist Elyakim Kislev found that it was more important to people who were not married than to married people to make their own decisions and to be free. When he focused on the happiest people, he found that the difference got bigger: it was even more important to the happiest single people than to the happiest married people to get to make their own decisions and to be free.[104]

Contributing to Our Communities

Community involvement is important to me. I volunteer at the local animal shelter. When a new shelter opened in my town, I commissioned an artist to create a pet-themed bike rack near the entrance. I also attend meetings of the neighborhood association and help out when I have time. After twelve years on a condo board, I've dialed back my involvement there, but I still like to stay involved. I belong to a grassroots transportation advisory group that gets involved in public projects in the early phases when it can make a difference. I had one job as a student supervisor for a high school foreign exchange program and got to help young people get the most out of their exchange experience (and in one case, rescue a student from a bad placement situation by keeping her at my house until I could find her a new host family). My current living situation is in a small intentional community, where we look after one another and share our limited resources. I recently delivered groceries to a family in our community who were all down with COVID. Oh, and I look after my tiny house host's elderly mom while they're snowbirding in Arizona and take over as community manager during that time as well.
—Kristin (fifty-five, Bellingham, Washington)

Kristin wasn't boasting when she said all that. I knew she had contributed to her community in all sorts of ways, and I asked her to pull it all together for me. I often think of her when I read studies showing the many ways that single people are particularly generous. For example, in the US, they volunteer more than married people do for community service organizations, cultural and sports groups, environmental organizations, health organizations, and just about every other kind of organization except religious groups.[105] In everyday life, they more often show up for friends, neighbors, and coworkers who need a ride, help with errands or work around the house, or moral and emotional support.[106] They contribute to the vitality of their cities and towns with their involvement in public events and civic groups.[107]

For Yolanda, a twenty-six-year-old from Washington, DC, volunteering is a way of life. As she shared, "Sometimes I think of how instead of starting to date as a teenager, I spent much of my time volunteering as a math and writing tutor. And I still volunteer today, over a decade later."

Maria, a fifty-two-year-old from Beverly, Massachusetts, said, "Volunteering for me is an integral part of who I am. When my daughter was younger I volunteered more in the schools (running science fairs at the elementary schools was important so they could see a woman who is an engineer). Now I do more with the green initiatives in my town. Each experience is meaningful in its own way."

When I taught a lifelong learning course on single life, a divorced woman proclaimed to the rest of the class that she hated being single. She did some volunteering, she said, but it was just a way to fill the time, and she found it boring and unfulfilling. Every night, she could not wait until it got late enough that she could finally justify just going to bed. It's different for the single at heart. One of the reasons they are drawn to single life is that they are in touch with who they really are and what they find fulfilling. Their volunteer work and their other contributions to their communities are not just things to do to pass the time; they are things they love to do.

Caring for Our People

It was an honor to help him.
—David (sixty-five, Austin, Texas), describing the last years
of his father's life, when he had Alzheimer's disease

The parents of single people may have once badgered them about marrying, but when those parents advance into their later years and need more and more help, they may be grateful to have grown children who are not coupled. Em, a forty-five-year-old from Cambridge, England, who told me she felt blessed to still have both parents, moved to be closer to them as they grew older. A US study of nearly fifty-five hundred parents who were sixty-five and older revealed that their single children were much more likely to provide the help they needed than their coupled children. That was true in the black families and the white ones, and it was true of both the sons and the daughters.[108]

It is not just parents who are finding single people at their doorsteps when they are most in need of help. When other people are sick, disabled, or elderly and need sustained help for at least three months, single people are more likely to provide that help, a study of more than nine thousand British adults showed.[109]

I'd like to say that the intensive care that single people provide is an unmitigated good thing, with no risks, but I'm not so sure. Helping can feel like an honor, as David said, and it can come from a place of deep, abiding love. But alongside that love, there can be other psychological dynamics. In her study of black middle-class singles with no children, University of Maryland sociologist Kris Marsh found that the women often felt obligated to help family members and people who were like family to them, even when it cost them financially, physically, or psychologically.[110] It is almost always financially riskier for a solo single person to take time off from work to help other people; they don't have a spouse who can pay the bills for them, and in the US, the Family and Medical Leave Act only covers time taken off to care for a spouse, parent, or child.

Sometimes single people are pressured into the role of the designated helper by other people's demeaning assumption that because they are single, they don't have a life. I've heard stories like that, but rarely from people who are single at heart. Like David, they are more likely to say that helping someone they cared about, even when that was difficult and went on for years, was their choice and their honor.

Helping other people while living with them, though, can be particularly challenging for the single at heart, who greatly value their freedom and solitude. A single woman from India emailed me about this. She is an only child who lives alone and loves being single. When she is home alone, she paints and creates music. She also has regular outings with her friends. In India, she told me, the concept of filial duty is very strong, and she has always been devoted to her parents. She calls them every day and has always visited them for a month or so, twice a year. This time, they were staying with her for a few months. It has worked out well in some ways. She has escorted them to doctors' appointments and taken them to interesting places they have enjoyed. But she no longer engages in her artistic pursuits because she needs absolute solitude for them. She still sees her friends occasionally, but now she feels a bit guilty about spending that time away from her parents. "I also feel like my home is not my own; they tend to take over and do things their way," she said. "I will be sad when they leave, but I will also be happy to have my house back."

The single at heart, including the woman from India, often talk about the people they help with deep love. Some of them have told me that of all the things they could do with their freedom, what they wanted most was to be there for the important people in their lives. Carla, a thirty-three-year-old from Essex, England, said that freedom means "spending as much time as I want with my parents and friends. This is particularly poignant to me as I lost my dad two and a half years ago, and if I'd had a serious partner in the year or so before, I'd not have been able to spend nearly as much time with Dad, and that time is so precious now."

In 2012 two scholars interviewed twenty-six Irish men and women who were between sixty-five and eighty-six years old and had never been married. Many of them had spent substantial portions of their adult lives caring for their parents or other relatives. Some of them described their caregiving with a touch of resentment as something they had to do. Others said they were happy to reciprocate the love and caring they had enjoyed as children. The difference was clear. The regretful helpers had wanted to marry. The happy helpers were happily single.[111]

There are exceptions, of course, especially when the demands of caring are particularly onerous, go on for a long time, or when the helper's relationship with the person they are helping is fraught. Iris, a sixty-five-year-old single mother in Portugal who shared that she was not the daughter her mother had always wanted, said, "It was not easy to care for my mother in the last ten years of her life, since she was still 'praying for me.'. . . On the other hand, taking care of my brilliant kid always made total sense to me."

People such as the single at heart who cherish their freedom and embrace individualistic values such as creativity, self-expression, and autonomy are at the cutting edge of global social change. A half-century of data from seventy-eight nations revealed that individualistic values and practices have been increasing in most countries around the world.[112] To some scholars and cultural commentators, those trends are troubling. They see individualistic people as self-centered types who just don't care about families, communities, or anyone but themselves. They urge us to exchange our "easy drift toward selfish autonomy for a cultivated embrace of self-discipline and communal responsibility."[113]

As my study of the single at heart suggests, though, those concerns are unwarranted. Findings from a study of 152 countries add further support, showing that people who are more individualistic—valuing autonomy, self-expression, and the pursuit of personal goals—are more generous. They are more likely to volunteer, help strangers, give to charity, support the humane treatment of animals, and donate blood, or even organs.[114] The social scientists who did the research do not know for sure why people who value freedom are more generous. One of them, Georgetown University professor Abigail Marsh, believes that one possibility is that "individualism boosts altruism by psychologically freeing people to pursue goals that they find meaningful—goals that can include things like alleviating suffering and caring for others."[115]

For the single at heart, individualism can be psychologically freeing in another way. Without the expectations of conventional coupling that a spouse, family, and maybe even in-laws are to be prioritized over all else, single people get to set their own priorities. Those priorities can include altruistic aspirations such as contributing to communities and caring for other people.

Choosing Our Spaces, Our Places, and Our Homes

When I left my childhood home, I moved into a house about a block away that my parents had purchased for my paternal grandfather to live in until his passing. I had such a treasure in that little house. It was mine entirely to decorate, to play my music as I wished, and to come and go from while going to college and working at the television station. I also learned how to take care of a house like that—making mistakes along the way, but learning. I was still near my beloved parents, but I was living alone for the first time in my life. My own actual space and place in the world. In every moment, I was able to be only the person I wanted to be and not compelled toward another person's vision or expectations.
—David (sixty-five, Austin, Texas)

Because we do not have a romantic partner to accommodate, the single at heart can, within the limits of our resources and opportunities, live however we wish. Because single life is not, for us, a matter of marking time until that one special person comes along, we don't put off buying a home if that's what we want to do and can afford, and we don't treat the places where we live as way stations, filling them with makeshift furniture and haphazard decor. Many of us attend lovingly to our living spaces, turning them into homes that comfort, energize, or inspire us and reflect who we really are.

As I will discuss in the chapter on solitude, more than half of the people who are clearly single at heart live alone. Sometimes that means living in an apartment or a neighborhood where, at least initially, we know no one else. But if we want the freedom and privacy of a place of our own, while living close to people we care about, we find ways to attain that. Kristin, for example, lives in a tiny house in a tiny house community.

In years of asking single people to share their fantasies about how they want to live, one of the most popular ones involves plotting with longtime friends, who may have scattered over the years, to reconvene in a place where they can all live near one another. Eleanor Wilkinson has studied single people in the UK who have no romantic partner, no children, and no desire to become coupled or have a conventional family. She described a group of five of those single people who had known each other for more than a decade and who made good on that fantasy. They moved to a small town where they all found places within walking distance of one another.[116]

In my research for *How We Live Now*, I interviewed two friends, both widows, who have homes of their own next door to each other. Another pair of friends, both divorced, each live in their own home on opposite ends of a duplex they bought together. Another single woman, Lucy, had no romantic partner, no kids, no living parents, and no relatives within an eight hundred-mile radius. What she did have was a lifetime of friends, and she created her own safe community for herself and six other lesbians. When she was forty-nine, she bought several acres of neglected land pocked with run-down buildings and transformed it into a lush landscape with rebuilt homes. She's been living there with her friends for decades.

Some people who are single at heart don't just want to live near the important people in their lives, they want to live under the same roof with them. Such was the case for Andrea (twenty-nine, New York City), who shared with me her passion for living with friends in college:

> Senior year of college I lived in a house of seven girls and
> seven guys, a bedroom to myself, people came and went as
> they pleased, did as they pleased. Sometimes I'd have a one-
> on-one deep conversation in the kitchen, some nights we'd

throw wild parties, some evenings we'd pile onto the couch and watch a show with rapt attention . . . it was a *dream*! I would love to live like that forever.

Andrea's fantasy of living with dear friends, enjoying fun times and intimate conversations, is shared by single people of every age. It is a dream that transcends continents and cultures. In the Community of Single People Facebook group, one story has been shared again and again, year after year. It inspires an outpouring of likes, loves, and covetous comments every time. The story is about seven women from China who had been friends for more than twenty years and had always fantasized about finding a place they could share once they were retired. Then they found it, an abandoned red brick house in a village set among verdant fields and rice paddies about an hour away from the city of Guangzhou in southeast China.[117]

The women pooled their money to buy the house, which they completely rebuilt into a bright, open, contemporary multistory mansion, with floor-to-ceiling windows, porches, and balconies. They share an enormous kitchen on the first floor and enjoy their own private bedrooms on the upper floors. Outside they built a tea pavilion and a swimming pool. They are not yet retired, but why wait? They already cook together and sing together, and just as Andrea dreamed, they gather in the living room to bask in the warmth of one another's company.

The single people who told me their tales of longing to live with other people usually had friends in mind. But a home and a life can be shared with any loving and compatible humans (and pets). In *Gay and Single . . . Forever?*, Steven Bereznai described a sixty-six-year-old gay man, Wayson, who "currently co-owns two houses, with two different families, one with his 'city family' and one with his 'country family.' In both cases they are a straight couple with one or more kids, and Wayson is their godfather. The houses aren't split up into apartments, they live together."[118]

· · ·

Now that I'm through with my workplace work, I'm moving to New Mexico where I can live among the natural environments of desert, mountains, and big skies with sunsets and sunrises that I can actually watch.

—David (sixty-five, Austin, Texas)

I've experienced love at first sight several times in my life. My most recent experience was eight years ago, when I was searching for a new place after the rent at my previous place slipped beyond my means. I walked into a small house with bright, open, airy rooms and big windows with a peak of the Pacific Ocean, and I just knew. This house would be my home, my new love. And it has been. I'm attached to it. I feel comfortable and secure when I am here, and I miss it when I am away. I'll only move if I have to.

It is wrong to describe single people as "unattached" because, as I will explain later, we often have secure attachments to the important people in our lives. But it is also wrong to think about attachments as something specific to other people. We can become lovingly attached in other ways—for example, to homes, countries or regions, communities, and places such as that special coffee shop that feel like our home away from home. The single at heart use our freedom to honor all of our attachments.

Pursuing a Meaningful Life

In the year 2000, I moved from Virginia to California for what was supposed to be a one-year sabbatical at the University of California at Santa Barbara. Before then, I had just visited briefly, and I only knew people superficially as colleagues I had met at conferences. But I figured, it was only a year so it wouldn't matter if I didn't like it.

I loved it. I could tell you that I was smitten by the awe-inspiring beauty, the weather that is at least as amazing as it appears in the movies, my warm and brilliant colleagues who were becoming friends, and a university adorned with flags honoring their Nobel Laureates. All that is true, but it felt deeper. I had found my home.

A few weeks before I needed to start planning my return to Virginia, I was walking the beach with a friend, telling her how much I wished I could stay. To which she replied, "So, stay."

Staying would entail big changes in my life, including leaving behind a friendship network decades in the making, a home that I owned, and a tenured professorship at the University of Virginia. At UCSB, I was a visiting professor, an unpaid position. Financially, it would be a huge risk. I did it anyway.

People who don't know me very well have pointed out that it would have been easier if I had a spouse who could pay the bills for a while. I've always given the same answer. I would not want to ask a partner, no matter how loving or how willing, to move across the country and cover for me financially so I could do what I wanted.

Really, though, I never wanted a romantic partner, so I never did that psychological arithmetic. My mental calculations were about meaning. My move to California was a turning point. I committed to a new place and a new mental space. I was growing ever more passionate about my work on single people. Within a few years, I would (mostly) leave behind my expertise on the psychology of lying and detecting lies I had spent many years developing and devote the rest of my life to the study and practice of single life.

Reimagining Holidays

I feel free to spend holidays and vacations as I wish. I don't feel obligated to "go home" to repetitive and uninspiring holiday "traditions."
—Evan (forty, San Francisco, California)

Growing up, I loved traditional, repetitive holiday celebrations. For Thanksgiving, my parents, grandparents, aunts, uncles, siblings, and cousins all gathered around a big table that groaned under the weight of the turkey and all the trimmings, a feast that was served up only after we had all devoured a first course of ravioli and meatballs.

One of my cousins had stayed single her whole life, and because of her presence at the Thanksgiving table, I was rarely bored. Unlike the rest of us, for whom the dinner was our first and only event of the day, Karen had already been out and about, often at a football game, and she regaled us with stories of the antics on and off the field. She was a high school principal who was beloved by her students. She retired many years ago, and to this day, her students are still finding her on Facebook and telling her how much she meant to them.

If all my relatives had lived forever and stayed in Pennsylvania, maybe I would still be heading back there each November. Over time, though, even when the traditional celebration was still an option, other possibilities intrigued me. When I was living in Charlottesville, I was part of a cooking club that lasted for a decade. The food was fascinating—we chose a different cuisine each time—and the conversation was too. One year, someone proposed a cooking club Thanksgiving. I declined. That was the first time I felt that by returning to my hometown for the kind of traditional family holiday that is celebrated, revered, and sentimentalized, I was missing out on something I may have enjoyed more.

> I had one of my best Christmas experiences on one of my cross-country road trips. I got stranded (due to a snowstorm) in a Walmart parking lot and ended up striking up a conversation and subsequent friendship with the only other person who was also stuck in the parking lot. We swapped travel stories for hours. It was just a fun, serendipitous set of circumstances. I think that I am flexible, adaptable, and open-minded enough to be able to enjoy myself and make connections with people anywhere, even under unfavorable conditions like being stuck in a Walmart parking lot. —Mary (thirty-three, Buffalo, New York)

In response to my question, "How do you feel about holidays and vacation times?" Yolanda (twenty-six, Washington, DC), Harini (forty-seven, New York), Julie (forty-four, Raleigh, North Carolina), and

Eva (forty-four, London, England) all responded with some variation of "Love them!" Claudia (sixty-nine, Washington, DC) added, "Thanksgiving 2018, I spent eight days in Paris. Had a great time!"

Carmela, a forty-four-year-old from Nayarit, Mexico, has been treated like family by several different families who live near her. She visits each of them on holidays. Sophia (fifty-seven, England) likes to hang out with her kids on holidays. Plus, she added, "every day is a vacation day when you work part time." Beth, a fifty-six-year-old from San Mateo, California, spends holidays with her father; vacations are for traveling or staycations. Sonya (forty-seven, Parkersburg, West Virginia) said, "My 'blood' family meets only twice a year, for Thanksgiving and a family reunion. I'm glad to see them. I'm also glad to see them go."

There is no one single at heart way of vacationing or spending a holiday. That's one of the joys of single life. We have the freedom to explore options, create our own traditions, or embrace the opportunity to be completely and blissfully alone.

Curating Our Everyday Lives

I like going to bed when I want, no one interrupting my sleep, waking up when I want. Eating what I want, when I want. Exercising when I want, how I want. I don't have to feel guilty about wanting to do something on my own. There are no interruptions or distractions while I am reading or meditating.
—Andrea (twenty-nine, New York City)

Making the most of the freedom of single life does not have to mean traveling the world, becoming a rock star, or devoting years of your life to the care of a parent or cherished relative or friend. Sometimes contentment and fulfillment come from the small stuff, such as arranging our schedules, our homes, and the structures of our everyday lives just the way we like them.

My uncle Joe spent his whole adult life married to a woman who loved shopping, visiting relatives, going on day trips, telling stories, and laughing. He was a quieter and calmer person, but it didn't matter; he adored her and was happy to be as busy as she wanted to be. When she died, he was bereft. A few months afterward, I asked him what his life was like. He said, "I get up. I make my coffee, make my breakfast. Then I sit quietly and enjoy it. When I'm good and ready, I move on to the next part of my day." He was still grieving, and he never would have identified as single at heart, but he did a very single at heart thing by finding solace in a peaceful, unhurried routine that suited his temperament.

I worry that single people sometimes feel pressured to live great big impressive and hugely magnanimous lives, almost as if they think they have to compensate for their single status. Coupled people, in contrast, rarely feel that they have to justify their lives; just being coupled provides automatic legitimacy. As "Onely" blogger Christina Campbell argued in "Sitting on the couch in stained sweatpants: Is it cool?", "A relatively sedentary single person living a non-mind-blowing life is as respect-worthy as the single person hammering fenceposts in Namibia. Activities don't matter—what's important is your inner moral compass and kindness to others."[119]

Who Gets to Enjoy All That Freedom?

It can be annoying that you have to do everything yourself—
no splitting the bills, having help with the lawn work, etc.
But I make a good living, so I can outsource and Amazon Prime
now delivers cough medicine and chicken soup when I'm sick.
This new world of automation and convenience have made it
especially easy to be single. It would be very hard if I didn't
have the resources to live this life, and I can see
why some people marry for security.
—Donna (forty-nine, Seattle, Washington)

To fully enjoy the freedom that the single at heart prize takes resources and opportunities that not everyone has. Living the most unfettered version of the single life is more of a stretch for people who are struggling economically or have caring obligations, disabilities, or challenges to their physical or mental health.

The obstacles are not just personal. In many societies, there are institutional impediments such as laws, policies, and practices that benefit only people who are married. Single people are systematically disadvantaged—that's singlism. Singlism can be exacerbated by many of the other intersecting "isms," such as racism, sexism, classism, ageism, and ableism. Embracing single life can also be difficult in places where very few people are single or live alone, or where family life is deeply valued and single life is not.

And yet, as I will show, even under the most trying circumstances, many people embrace their single lives. They do so as an act of being true to themselves, of living the life that is best for them, even if they wish it were not so daunting to do so.

In theory, anyone can identify as single at heart. No one needs wealth, health, or any other advantage in order to *want to* fashion a life that does not have a romantic partner at its center. In theory, it should not just be the most privileged people who see solitude as sweet, who like being the deciders, and who see single life as their most authentic and meaningful life.

And in fact, privilege is not a prerequisite for identifying as single at heart and living single joyfully and unapologetically. On the single at heart quiz, people from all over the world, and not just those from the wealthiest nations or the most individualistic ones, scored as single at heart. On average, people who qualified as single at heart had no more income than those who were not single at heart, were no more likely to be employed, and were only slightly more educated.

Faced with personal or more systematic obstacles to living single, many people who are single at heart nonetheless persist in living the most expansive version of single life they can manage. Single life is their most authentic, meaningful, and fulfilling life, so they do not give it up lightly. Living under lockdown for months on end during the pandemic, for example, did not motivate them to give it all up and succumb to coupling.

Caring obligations can curb our freedoms, as the woman who emailed me from India explained, but sometimes caring for others is what we choose to do with our freedom. Needing care can be constraining too, yet people with devastating injuries and life-threatening illnesses, for example, have continued to live fulfilling single lives, even in the context of health care systems that are far more accommodating to people who are not single.

Many policies and practices need to change to create a more just and more welcoming world for single people. In the meantime, the single at heart are persisting in embracing their single lives, despite the obstacles, as the next two stories illustrate.

• • •

I haven't consistently associated singlehood with freedom.
My freedom always carries severe constraints based on what my sparkly
blue manual wheelchair and I need to be successful at a particular
moment in a particular place. My living spaces are arranged to best
support my physical abilities and where, when, and whether I travel
depends upon the kindness of others. When I can't find a job that meets
my disability modification and accommodation requirements,
I have no job at all. If I'm always going to be dependent, at least to
some degree, then why don't I become the most socially valued kind of
dependent, like Cinderella? For me, my cherished singlehood
is my opportunity to redefine my relationship to independence every day
in order to best honor my body, my mind, and my spirit.
I'm proud of my kinship with the people who have fought for the
freedoms that allow me to choose singlehood. In their honor,
I try to be my most vibrant, joyful self, someone who brings
a loving presence to all kinds of relationships.
—Jill Summerville, PhD

Marginality, bell hooks argued, is "much more than a site of deprivation." Instead, "it offers the possibility of radical perspectives from which to see and create, to imagine alternatives, new worlds."[120] Jill Summerville has reimagined freedom. Nothing stops her from being her "most vibrant, joyful self, someone who brings a loving presence to all kinds of relationships."

People who stay single have often been stereotyped as not fully adult, because we do not meet the conventional milestone of getting married. The single at heart are rewriting what it means to be an adult, as we create meaningful and fulfilling life paths beyond the confines of conventional family life. From a disability perspective, people such as Jill are showing us how to think even more deeply about these issues. In an essay she wrote for the website of Unmarried Equality, an organization that stands for equality and fairness for unmarried Americans, she pointed out that "someone who is chronologically an adult might need assistance with physical tasks, such as walking, eating, or getting into bed, [and] never obtain a driver's license. . . . In 'disability time,' all of these people are successfully 'adulting.'"[121]

Other devalued groups have also contributed in deeply significant ways to our understanding of what it could mean to live a fulfilling single at heart life. For example, queer communities and communities of color have been at the forefront of creating and appreciating families of choice.[122] Indigenous communities show us how to think about relationships in the most expansive ways, as when we see ourselves as connected not just to other living people, but to ancestors, spiritual figures, pets, and the natural world.[123] And as sociologist Kris Marsh has shown, black women have been trailblazers in forging fulfilling single lives.[124]

In her contribution to an anthology of essays by women who are happily single, Bama, age sixty, counted her blessings. "I have a lovely nest of a home where I can freely sing, dance, laugh, or weep," she shared. "Another blessing this life has given me is the opportunity to live in harmony with nature. I wake up to the chirping of sparrows and the soulful sound of the cuckoo . . . My single womanhood has helped me tremendously to be a duty-conscious, responsible, and devoted teacher . . . I looked upon all my students as my own children and cared for their well-being."[125]

Summing up, Bama added, "I feel proud of my life alone. I think of it as a life well lived. It has been an immensely meaningful and satisfying life."

Bama sounds a lot like many of the other people who shared their life stories with me. What it took for her to live single, though, was entirely different. Bama lives in India, where only 1 percent of women stay single. She is a Dalit, a member of a stigmatized caste. When she wanted to live alone, no one would rent her a house. Eventually, a Dalit couple let her rent a small room in their home, but they subjected her to what she described as "indescribable humiliations and restrictions." Then, with no warning and for no stated reasons, they ordered her to vacate immediately. Next, she took on the enormous challenge of building a small home on her own. She succeeded, but for that, she was derided rather than celebrated. Out loud, in front of her, people made comments such as, "She is wasting her money building this house just for a single person," and, "She should get married; otherwise, she will be sitting in her empty house like a lonely owl."[126]

Bama was assigned to work at a remote village school, and to stay late at night for school functions, even when that meant walking home alone along dark and dangerous roads. She was told that she had to cover those duties since she had no family responsibilities; it would be too difficult for the married women.

The sexual harassment Bama endured was relentless. She was even ridiculed for needing surgery to have fibroids removed. A rumor was started in her village that she had an abortion, not a hysterectomy.

Bama said that she chose to be single. I wonder whether, under the same circumstances, I would feel that I had no choice but to marry. Bama's story is an important reminder that "choosing" to be single is not merely a matter of accessing your authentic self and embracing the single at heart person that you find there. Social, cultural, religious, and structural barriers—even less onerous ones than those faced down by Bama—can be formidable. Her story is also an inspiration, showing what some people are willing to do to claim their single lives even under the most daunting circumstances.

Advice For the Single at Heart

Have you been able to learn and grow, pursue the work and passions you find most meaningful, live where and how you want, decide for yourself how to manage your money, contribute to your community in the ways that matter most to you, or be there for the people you care about? Those are genuine accomplishments that deserve to be appreciated and applauded.

Share the experiences you've found most joyful and meaningful. They are at least as interesting as the stories coupled people tell about their partners, and maybe a lot less predictable. Appreciate that you get to choose a job that is for you and not to support a partner or fund pieces of a life that you don't want or need.

Have you felt stymied in your efforts to live your most fulfilling single life by laws and policies that disadvantage single people? Remember that your difficulties are not about being single, but about the ways in which societies deliberately cater to married people and their families and marginalize people who are single.

Because you will be supporting yourself, educate yourself about financial planning so you will always be able to afford your adventures, passions, caregiving, and contributions to your community.

For Our Allies

Ask single people what they love to do, what they enjoy most about their work, whether there's something they've done that makes them feel especially proud. Celebrate their accomplishments. Keep in mind that having freedom is not the same as having all the time in the world. Single people who live alone don't have another person who helps with the grocery shopping, the cooking, or any of the other household chores. Remember too that their life pursuits are just as important as those of coupled people; there is no reason to expect them to cover for others at work or have last dibs on vacation times. Guard against the stereotype that connects freedom to selfishness and remember the studies that show that more freedom often brings with it more selfless actions.

For People Who Are Intrigued by Single Life, But Have Concerns

Think about all the things you've always wanted to do that you have never gotten to. Would you be more likely to do those things if you were single?

Do you love the freedom afforded by single life, but feel guilty about that? You should never feel guilty about living your most authentic, joyful, meaningful, and fulfilling life. Living inauthentically is the real risk, both for you and the other people in your life.

4

Solitude

Waking up alone I feel no sense of loneliness, no wish to have someone
to talk to. The aloneness feels inherent, a trait rather than an event. I
can happily stay alone for days on end—writing, gardening, exercising,
walking, reading, watching movies. I have a degree of privacy, quiet, and
time to reflect that's inconsistent with a shared life. Without that ability
to contemplate, to be rather than to do, on a regular basis, I would not
enjoy life nearly as much as I do. I wouldn't be the same person.

—Joan (seventy-three, Newark, Delaware)

Liking her time alone is not just some random fun fact about Joan, akin
to her favorite color or flavor of ice cream. It is, as she said, inherent. It is
defining. It is necessary. Ketaki (thirty-four, Manipal, India) agreed. Without
alone time, she said, "I don't feel complete."

We who are single at heart share a kinship with the people Fenton Johnson
calls "solitaries." In *At the Center of All Beauty: Solitude and the Creative Life*, Johnson
describes solitaries as those "who are choosing to live alone or who deliberately
carve out periods of solitude from otherwise conventionally coupled lives."[127] He
said that they experience their solitude "not as tragedy or bad luck or loneliness,
but as an integral and necessary aspect of who they were."[128]

If you could watch those of us who are single at heart on a secret camera
that follows us everywhere, all day, every day, you would find that some
of us spend a lot of time alone. You would see that many of our pursuits,
when we are in our homes and when we are out and about, are solitary
ones. If you are good at reading body language, you would probably also
realize that we are comfortable in our solitude. We rarely feel lonely when we
are alone.

That would come as a surprise to all those who lean on stereotypes for their understanding of single life. When Wendy Morris and I asked participants in our research to tell us what came to mind when they thought about single people, and they could say anything at all, one in every six said that single people were lonely. When we instead asked people to tell us what came to mind when they thought about married people, only one person in 552 said that married people were lonely.[129]

I expected solitude to be important to people who are single at heart. But I had no idea just how fundamental it would be to just about every person who identifies as single at heart, or how much the single at heart would cherish their alone time, until I started tallying the data. In the single at heart quiz, I asked, "When you think about spending time alone, what thought comes to mind first?" The alternatives were "Oh, no, I might be lonely!" and "Ah, sweet solitude." Of those who were definitely single at heart, an astonishing 98 percent chose sweet solitude. Of those who identified as clearly *not* single at heart, a majority, 59 percent, instead worried about feeling lonely.

When I asked the forty-one single at heart people who shared their life stories how important, if at all, it was to have time to themselves, every last one of them said that it was important. Some used all caps to type things like VERY, EXTREMELY, and HUGELY. Three said it was like breathing.

The distinction between loneliness and solitude has echoed across decades of writings about solitude. In May Sarton's 1965 book *Mrs. Stevens Hears the Mermaids Singing*, she wrote, "Loneliness is the poverty of self; solitude is the richness of self."[130] In Alice Koller's 1990 book *The Stations of Solitude*, she wrote, "Being solitary is being alone well: being alone luxuriously immersed in doings of your own choice, aware of the fullness of your own presence rather than the absence of others."[131] In *Alone Together*, an anthology of essays about the pandemic, Anna Quinn noted, "They're so different, loneliness and solitude, one is something missing, the other something found."[132]

When I try to figure out why those of us who are single at heart are so enamored of single life, nothing—except, perhaps, our cherishing of freedom—seems more significant than our love of the time we have to ourselves. Because we experience our alone time as richness and fullness, as something found rather than something missing, solitude doesn't scare us, and loneliness does not plague us.

Our experience of solitude is unspoiled by some of the concerns so often attached to aloneness. Compared to other single people who also like spending time alone but want to be coupled, our enjoyment of our alone time is not undermined by the uneasy sense that we should be out there looking for a romantic partner. Compared to coupled people, we do not worry that we should cut short the time we want to ourselves to be with our partner.

Our love of solitude has already sustained us through a pandemic. It also inoculates us against the stories designed to frighten us into coupling. We had better hurry up and find someone, otherwise we will end up alone? That's not a threat. We like spending time alone. And we don't buy into the narrow-minded view that without a romantic partner at the center of our lives, we are alone in the world.

> ~~One is the loneliest number.~~
> **Fixed it!**
> *One is a whole number.*

We Like Companionship Too

Everyone has an optimal balance of the time they like to have to themselves and the time they like to spend socializing with other people. The single at heart tilt toward preferring proportionately more solitude, but some of us cherish plenty of companionship too. Joan, who described her love of solitude so movingly at the beginning of this chapter, also said this: "I'm often among the last to leave a party, and I feel disappointed when I'm having lunch or dinner with friends and someone looks at their watch and starts the exodus."

Our preferred balance of solitude and companionship is probably shaped by our culture, backgrounds, and upbringing, and it can change over time as our lives unfold. In my young adult years, when I was a university professor, I was perfectly happy to have just one day a week all to myself. Now, as a retiree approaching seventy, I'm perfectly happy when I have a social event scheduled for just one day a week.

What is special about solitude to the single at heart is not the amount of time we spend alone, or our preferred balance of solitude and companionship, but how we experience our alone time. We love it. That's not incompatible with loving other people and enjoying fulfilling relationships. Research shows that people who like spending time alone are no less likely to have positive, high-quality relationships with other people.[133] In fact, for the single at heart, we are probably better friends, more attentive to and engaged with the people in our lives, because we take our full measure of solitude. The time we have to ourselves makes us feel happy, healthy, and whole.

Our Role Models

When Andriette was sixty, she had already run eighty-five marathons, including twenty-four consecutive Boston Marathons, and she was profiled in *Runner's World* magazine. Andriette told the magazine that when she was in school, she was a bookworm who worked in the library. Reading and reflection continue to be important to her. She has a collection of more than three hundred books about running. At the local college where she teaches, her favorite course is "Running, Reading, and Reflecting."

Solitude seems to be an important component of her running life. Sometimes she runs alone in the wee hours, carrying a flashlight and looking for coins, which she collects all year and then donates to an animal shelter. When she drives to marathons, sometimes she stays overnight with friends or family, but more often she sleeps in her car.

She enjoys companionship too. Her secret weapon, she told *Runner's World*, is a cheering section that awaits her at the 22.5-mile mark when she runs near the city where she once lived.

Danielle, a fifty-one-year-old from Minneapolis, has run with Andriette and named her as her role model:

> She's the most like me, or at least who I want to be—friend-ly, free-spirited, fun. I met her when I separated after less than five years of marriage and moved back to the Midwest. When we gather to do long runs, trail runs, or track work-outs together, we talk mostly about running, far less about work or family. This shift in focus buoyed me as I put my life back together. It felt right to shape my goals around the things I loved to do, places I wanted to see, and optimizing my health and fitness, rather than the traditional American dream of career-house-spouse-pets-children.
>
> A few years ago, Andriette showed up to a Duluth race with a handsome running buddy. "He's a friend," she con-fided. "I don't date."

What We Get Out of Our Solitude

I feel the most at peace, the most relaxed, the most joyous, when I am
by myself or just with my cat. I love doing things on my own—
seeing movies, going out to dinner, reading, watching TV, traveling.
—Acadia (thirty-six, Melbourne, Australia)

Acadia's description, like Joan's (quoted at the beginning of this chapter), exudes calm. Research shows that people who like their time alone feel especially calm and relaxed when they have spent time in solitude.[134] People who are single at heart also report that they are rarely bored when they are on their own. As Carmela (forty-four, Nayarit, Mexico) said, "I can last a long time with myself without getting bored."

The experience of spending time alone is very different for those who don't like it, psychologists have shown.[135] They're bored. They're lonely. They don't know what to do with themselves. They descend into rumination, obsessing about how awful they are or how terribly other people have treated them. With no one else around, they aren't even interested in the kinds of pursuits they ordinarily find meaningful. Instead, they scroll endlessly through social media, not because they are truly interested in anything they find there, but because any distraction is better than sitting with their own thoughts. Sometimes they do the things other people expect or want them to do, even though no one is monitoring them.

What's distracting for me is not my own thoughts, but the presence of other people. When other humans are around, they steal a sliver of my mind, even if they are just quietly going about their own business. They are in my awareness. I can focus better when I am totally alone. I'm more productive. I can delve deeper into my studies, writing, and thinking.

Solitude is good for breadth as well as depth. While couples may lock eyes with one another and feel deeply connected, the single at heart treasure what they see and experience when another person is not blocking their view. In *Alone Time*, Stephanie Rosenbloom wrote, "When you're not sitting across from someone, you're sitting across from the world."[136] She was writing about dining alone, but I think she would concur with Fenton Johnson's more expansive rendering: "In solitude, the world, and not another individual, becomes the focus of one's ardent and respectful heart."[137]

Being alone, for people such as the single at heart, is liberating. It frees them to cultivate their creativity. Jennifer (forty-five, Denver, Colorado) said that she is "more creative and inspired when I have time alone." Sara Maitland, author of *How to Be Alone*, believes that solitude is especially conducive to creativity. "Creating something yourself, of your own, uniquely, requires a kind of personal freedom, a lack of inhibition, a capacity not to glance over your shoulder at the opinions of others."[138] I think Marie, a forty-six-year-old from Northern California, was describing something similar when she said that she appreciated that "'space' where access to my inner world is seamless. I can reside there uninterrupted."

Solitude can be a sacred space for spirituality and communion with the divine. It is also a special place for communing with ourselves. We feel more authentic when we are alone than when we are with other people, research shows.[139] With time for self-reflection, we can better understand how we really feel and what we really want. People who find meaning in solitude are especially likely to live mindfully in their everyday lives, attuned to moment-to-moment feelings regardless of whether other people are around.[140]

Solitude is our mental health spa, our place of peace. Carmela said, "I am a better person when everything is calm." Spending time alone protects us from the unpleasant persons we could become without it. It is, as Carla (thirty-three, Essex, England) said, "absolutely essential in order for me not to be grumpy, miserable, and downright horrible to be around!" It also allows us to do better than just not being grumpy. Again, it was Sara Maitland who understood this: "The joy of long periods of solitude has also increased my joy in non-solitude: I love my children, my friends, my colleagues as much as ever, and I attend to them better when I am with them—and enjoy them more."[141]

Positive attitudes toward solitude have been linked to good mental health. People who experience alone time the way the single at heart do—they are more creative or more focused when they are alone, and they enjoy having time to themselves in a pleasant environment—report better physical and psychological health, more positive feelings and fewer negative ones.[142]

Solitude can be sublime, but it can also be pedestrian. We who are single at heart appreciate the freedom it gifts us to listen to music, watch TV, surf the net, play online games, putter around the house, go out for a run, do errands, and just go about our daily routines.

Solitude is an acquired taste.[143] —*Washington Post*

Fixed it!

Solitude is comfort food for the soul.

The Personality Profiles of People Who Savor Their Solitude

Solitude is the wealth and coin of positive singleness.
—David (sixty-five, Austin, Texas)

When I first analyzed the data from the quiz I created, and learned that just about everyone who identified as single at heart regarded their time alone as sweet solitude, and then found that all forty-one people who shared their life stories did the same, I thought I knew just what that meant: we are all introverts.

Well, not quite. I didn't ask about introversion in the quiz, but I did ask the forty-one people who shared their life stories. They disproportionately identified as introverts. Some, however, said they were ambiverts who have both introverted and extroverted tendencies. A few considered themselves extroverts.

What was I not yet understanding about the personalities of people who enjoy their time alone? Thuy-vy T Nguyen and her colleagues have been studying the psychology of solitude for years. They too wanted to learn about the kinds of people who spend time alone because they enjoy it and value it and not just because they want to avoid other people.

In four studies, they recruited people to keep diaries of how they were spending their time, who they were with, and how they were feeling, day after day, for up to two weeks.[144] The participants completed a series of personality tests. The introverts were those who tended to describe themselves as quiet, reserved, and sometimes shy, and not as outgoing, sociable, or talkative.

The researchers discovered that introversion had little to do with cherishing solitude. The people who were outgoing, sociable, and talkative were no less likely to enjoy their own company and value having time to themselves than those who were quiet and reserved. You can be outgoing, talkative, and energetic and still enjoy spending time alone.

Instead, what mattered in study after study was authenticity. The people who were true to themselves were the ones who sought out solitude because they valued it and enjoyed their own company. On the personality tests, the authentic people tended to agree with statements such as "My actions are congruent with who I really am," and, "My whole self stands behind the important decisions I make." They are people who resist the pressure to feel or behave in particular ways. They tend to disagree with statements such as "I believe certain things so that others will like me" and "I do things in order to avoid feeling bad about myself."

Living your life authentically, in accordance with who you really are, and doing so despite all the norms, expectations, and pressures to live a coupled life instead, is true single at heart territory. Nguyen's diary studies of solitude show that people who are authentic seek out solitude and then get a lot out of it.

When Joan said that her solitude feels inherent, and without it, she wouldn't be the same person, I think she was telling us in her own way how authenticity matters. Mary (thirty-three, Buffalo, New York) expressed something similar when she said, "I feel most comfortable and most true to myself when I am alone."

But why should people who are true to themselves like solitude more and get more out of it? I think it is because when you are alone, you are face to face with just one person: yourself. If you are living an inauthentic life, that's uncomfortable. Alone with your thoughts, you obsess about what you don't like about yourself. You engage in mindless "doom scrolling" because it is a distraction from facing your phony self.

In Chapter 2 I shared stories from people who were miserable when they tried living the coupled life that was expected of them. They broke free of their misery and experienced true joy once they recognized and embraced their single at heart identity.

I'm not saying that we who are single at heart never find anything to dislike when we look inside ourselves. Nor am I saying we never experience misery, pain, anxiety, grief, or any other disturbing feelings. Of course we do. But with regard to decisions about coupling, any dissatisfaction with ourselves is not exacerbated by trying to live someone else's version of a good life instead of our own. Our distress can be brought on by all sorts of experiences and psychological dynamics, but living inauthentically, in some fundamental way, is not one of them.

What matters to our experience of solitude is not just what we see in ourselves when we look closely, but also our attitude toward self-examination. Do we welcome it or resist it? The solitude studies showed that the people who enjoyed their time alone were curious about themselves. On the personality tests, they tended to agree with statements such as, "I am interested in why I act the way I do."[145]

People who are self-reflective not only enjoy their alone time more, but they also appreciate the purest experiences of solitude. Lots of people who like being alone feel contented while reading, dipping into social media, or watching movies. People who are curious about themselves also feel comfortable just sitting in silence.[146]

Nguyen believes that people who are true to themselves and curious about their own reactions have an approach to life that is characterized by "taking interest in every bit of your experience."[147] I noticed something similar in the stories the single at heart shared with me. They seem to be savorers, who notice and appreciate even the small pleasures of everyday life. When I asked what makes her happy, Ginny (fifty-nine, Ontario, Canada) said, "I love the blue of the blue jay at the feeder right now. I love how Yo-Yo Ma recovered when his cello slipped while he was playing it. I love the sound of whip-poor-wills. I love the spiders in my kitchen, the birds at my feeders, my cats sleeping under their blankets."

Eva (forty-four, London, England) said, "There is beauty and happiness everywhere," then unfurled a long list, including, for example, "cold, sunny walk in the park, the crunchy noise of leaves, deer all around me, and hot, strong coffee in my hand."

The authenticity and curiosity that characterize people who relish their time alone is a remarkable repudiation of the damning stereotypes of them. In *How to Be Alone*, Sara Maitland bemoaned that people who exercise their freedom to be alone are regarded as "'sad or mad or bad.' Or all three at once."[148] In *Party of One: The Loners' Manifesto*, Anneli Rufus observed that people who like being alone are often smeared as criminals, crazies, haters, and outcasts.[149] Some people who spend a lot of time alone really are troubled. But they are not the people who want to be alone. They yearn to be coupled or to be included by other people, but instead they are ignored or rejected.

One more personality characteristic meaningfully separates people who like spending time alone from those who do not: they aren't very neurotic.[150] They are not particularly tense, moody, or inclined to worry a lot. Once again, embracing solitude for positive reasons is part of a profile of good mental health.

For people with low levels of neuroticism, just thinking about being alone can be motivating. In a series of studies, the psychologist Liad Uziel put participants in a mindset of being alone by asking them to complete the sentence, "When I am by myself, I . . . " He also created a social mindset by asking them to complete a different sentence, "When I am in the company of others, I . . . " The people who were not neurotic had at least as much willpower, if not more, when they thought about being by themselves compared to thinking about being with others. They were more willing to stand in a long line or read an entire boring book. Challenged with difficult anagrams, they spent more time on them and solved more of them. They sound like the single at heart people who told me that they are more productive when they are alone and that they rarely get bored.

Our Solitude Is Precious, So We Protect It

Author and essayist Meghan Daum wrote that some of the men she had dated were "interesting and smart . . ." "But," she added, "they were still no match for the solace of my apartment and the familiar rhythms of my own company. I couldn't imagine going home with any of them, partly because there's nothing I like better than going home by myself."[151]

Those of us who live alone have a lot of control over our solitude. We can decide if and when we want to welcome people into our homes, and for how long. It is more challenging when we are away.

When I lived in Charlottesville, Virginia, one of the highlights of my summers was renting a beach house for a week or two in Duck, North Carolina, a tiny town in the Outer Banks as adorable as its name. One year I rented the house with friends. They are wonderful, fun people, and I loved the idea of vacationing with them. But I didn't want to spend all of my time with them. I knew that some of the time, I would just want to be by myself.

I agonized about how to tell them that. It just seemed so weird, so unfriendly. Yet it had nothing to do with them. I wouldn't want to spend an entire week or two with anyone, sharing the home, the meals, the beach time, the walks, and everything else. The shared life that so many couples treasure is just the sort of life I would never want, not even for a short time, not even with friends I adored.

In subsequent years I decided to rent the house myself. That way I could invite people to join me on some of the days and have the others to myself. One year I saved the first day for myself and invited my parents to come after that. As I was settling in that first night and luxuriating in having a big, beautiful beach house to myself, a car pulled up in the driveway. My parents decided to surprise me and come early.

The next year I invited friends to join me for all except the last few days. The night before they were scheduled to leave, one of them asked to stay the rest of the time. She just didn't understand why I'd want a few days to myself.

I wish I knew at the time—and I wish my friends and family knew—that other people guard their precious solitude as devotedly as I do. From the life stories that people shared with me I learned that this is not at all uncommon among people who are single at heart.

Ginny (fifty-nine, Ontario, Canada) told me that when she is planning a vacation with other people, "Up front I let them know there would be times when I would need to go off on my own." She didn't seem to struggle with that the way I did. Carla (thirty-three, Essex, England), who now lives alone but used to live with friends, said, "Any time I live or stay with other people, my own room is a minimum requirement to keep me from quickly going insane."

Some people come up with strategies to secure the alone time they crave. Beth (fifty-six, San Mateo, California) stays in bed longer when she is visiting friends or vacationing with them. Carla said, "When I did live with people, and when I stay with Mum at Christmas, I retreat into books and use a firm system of closing my door as a signal I need some alone time, and/or go for a drive by myself."

Where Loneliness Finds Us

The loneliest of us are not necessarily those of us who are actually alone but rather those of us trying our hardest not to be alone.[152]
—Michael Cobb, *Single: Arguments for the Uncoupled*

People who are single at heart do feel lonely sometimes, but that tends to happen when they are not single or not living alone. "I began to feel very lonely. I had no time to myself and had no friends of my own," Kendra, a sixty-nine-year-old from San Francisco, California, told me. She was describing a time when she was married.

Ketaki (thirty-four, Manipal, India) said, "I began living alone for the first time in July 2019. I felt so happy. I used to feel lonely during my PhD days, despite living with roommates. I feel free and not lonely at all when I live alone."

The single at heart value authenticity not just in ourselves, but also in the other people in our lives. Marie (forty-six, Northern California) said she sometimes experiences loneliness "in large crowds or even apparent 'intimate' gatherings when the fellowship feels forced, fake, hostile, manipulated, passive-aggressive, or judgmental." After a while small talk can feel lonely and boring too. Some of us are just not very good at that.

Alone in Public

I travel all over the world without a companion, eat wherever I want
to, and go to social events or public events by myself without a second
thought, whether I know anyone who'll be there or not. That was never a
problem for me, since I never felt a need to organize my life around what
people I'd never seen before and would never see again might think.
—Joan (seventy-three, Newark, Delaware)

Joan isn't letting other people's possible judgments of her get inside her head and dissuade her from doing the things she loves, even when that means doing them alone and in public. People who are single at heart are less likely to be bandied about by other people's opinions and expectations. If we are going to claim our love of being single instead of trying to downplay it, we almost have to have that kind of resilience, because we are sure to face the skepticism and dismissal of people who refuse to believe that anyone could really want to be single.

More typically, people do worry about being judged if they do fun things like going to restaurants or movie theaters by themselves. Marketing professors Rebecca K. Ratner and Rebecca W. Hamilton did research in the US, China, and India, and found that in all three places, people worried that if they went to a movie theater by themselves, they would be judged more harshly than if they went with friends.[153] If they did go on their own, they preferred times when the theater would be less crowded, presumably so fewer people would see them alone. Their fear was that other people would think they were alone because they don't have any friends. Showing up with other people makes a statement: "See, I do have friends!" I think that doing fun things on your own makes a bolder statement: "I'm comfortable on my own."

Check out the self-assurance in David's account of his practice of dining alone: "Eating out is my favorite form of entertainment. I have dined alone for decades and I've never had any problems or encountered any real hassles for doing it solo. It is easier, I think, for a confident man to just walk in and kind of own my presence in a restaurant."

David (sixty-five, Austin, Texas) isn't just OK with dining alone. It's his favorite fun thing to do. Mary (thirty-three, Buffalo, New York) said the same thing about travel:

> I absolutely love to travel alone. It is my favorite way to travel. There is nothing better than having the total freedom that it affords you. You can change the day's itinerary at a moment's notice, and do what you want when you want. You never have to adapt your plans to another person's preferences.

Kendra (sixty-nine, San Francisco, California) said, "Some things I actually prefer going alone to as I can then go at my own pace." Carla describes another advantage: "Doing stuff on my own is especially nice if it's something like a dance performance where I can really focus on what I'm seeing and experiencing rather than paying attention to my companion." In *Single & Happy: The Party of Ones*, J. Victoria Sanders said, "Except when I go to the theater with one or two of my introverted friends, I mostly really, really love being in a theater with no one sitting next to me fussing about popcorn or complaining about the previews and the ads or whatever."[154]

David, Mary, Kendra, Carla, and Victoria discovered on their own what research has shown to be true: some things are more fun to do alone, and more memorable too. They are also right about the psychology of the experiences. Other people can be a distraction, even when they are people we like and whose company we often enjoy.[155]

The social scientists who conducted that research are not denying that many leisure experiences are in fact more fun with other people. Neither are the single at heart. They key is to understand the difference:

> In college I was a film critic and instinctively knew to go
> alone to any screening in order to hear my own thoughts

and write a comprehensive review. I still approach outings that way: is this an experience to delve into my insular journey uninterrupted or something to share and merit discussion? Do I wish to go deep and get still with this or explore depth at a different level to bounce it back and forth with another/others' viewpoint? —Marie (forty-six, Northern California)

Table for one? It's not as bad as it sounds.[156] —*New York Times*
Fixed it!
Table for one? That sounds divine.

Our Homes Are Our Sanctuaries

I've always wondered why people think I'm sad to live alone
when all I feel is relief and peace when I return home.
—Liz (sixty, Washington, DC)

When I was in grade school I received a prize for being mediocre. My teacher was curating an exhibit of the artwork of students in different grades, and she chose examples of work that was outstanding as well as work that was "representative." For the assignment, we could draw anything we liked. I chose a scene from a drive my family took quite often to my grandparents' place, along a stretch of highway in northeastern Pennsylvania bordered by dense forests. Smack in the middle of a thicket of trees was a house. Just one house, all by itself. I was mesmerized by it. That's what I drew.

Except for a year of sharing an apartment in graduate school because it was all I could afford, I have lived alone my entire adult life. I hope I will be able to continue to do so until the day I die. For many people who are single at heart, living alone is not something to fear. It is something we yearn for and treasure if we attain it.

We don't need a place of our own in order to carve out some time and space for ourselves. No one does. Daz (thirty-eight, Northern England), who lives with his parents, told me that he has always had time and space for himself. When I interviewed people for *How We Live Now: Redefining Home and Family in the 21st Century*, I found that even people who lived in big, bustling households found ways to secure some solitude. They got up before everyone else, or went for walks, or took long baths, or staked out a shed in the backyard, or found a special place alongside a creek.

Nonetheless, people who are single at heart are drawn disproportionately to solo living. Of the thousands of people who took the single at heart quiz, 56 percent of those who scored as definitely single at heart lived alone. That's not a huge percent. It's nowhere near the 98 percent who see their time alone as sweet solitude. But it is more than half, and a lot more than the percentage of adults who typically live alone. In the US in 2020, for example, out of a population of 251.9 million adults age eighteen and older, 36.2 million lived alone. That's 14.4 percent. As a percentage of just those adults who were not married, 118.8 million, it was 30.5 percent.

Lots of people like having time to themselves, regardless of their relationship status or whether they live alone or with others. In a Pew Research Center survey of a representative sample of adults in the US, 85 percent said that it was very important or somewhat important to have some time completely alone.[157] And yet, many people reach their solitude surfeit long before the single at heart do.

The Australian author Donna Ward, in *She I Dare Not Name: A Spinster's Meditations on Life*, described her visit with a man who had children and grandchildren, but chose to live alone. "He said that in solitude life becomes vibrant, aflame, everything tastes more of itself." Ward was skeptical, so she asked:

> What about that moment at the end of a day when you come into this stillness, where everything is as it was when you left, and the heavy door closes behind you, and the Aga needs stoking, and the kale needs cooking, the candles light-ing—how is that moment for you?

Ah. Well, he said, you have found the chink in my armour of solitude.[158]

The single at heart don't have that chink. The stories people told me were filled with odes to coming home to their sanctuaries. That's the word that came up again and again when they talked about their homes: sanctuary. Carla said, "I love the sanctuary of my home and the peace that is always waiting for me there after a busy day." Peggy (sixty-seven, Atlanta, Georgia) effused about how much she loved "getting home from work and closing the door behind me! No constant drama or conflict. Cats and dogs sleeping on the bed. No specific meal times. Decorating my house like I love!" Ketaki (thirty-four, Manipal, India) said, "I am happiest when I come home to an empty house." Some people made it clear that they do enjoy socializing, but still, their sanctuary beckons. Amy, a forty-four-year-old from Frisco, Texas, for example, said, "I love spending time with family and friends, but I love even more coming home to my own house and having time to myself to regroup."

I do too. I also relish everything that dented that man's armor. I love finding everything exactly as I left it when the door closes behind me. It warms my heart to be the sole decider of what adorns and brightens my home. I find cooking relaxing—though it wouldn't be kale and I'd be delighted if some cleaning fairy swooped in afterward and tidied things up, then left without a word.

Over lunch a person I was just starting to get to know told me that she was mostly fine being single, but she missed coming home at the end of the day to a romantic partner who would ask about her day. I understand that among some who are contentedly coupled, that's one of their day-to-day pleasures.

Some of the rest of us, though, savor our freedom from that ritual. In *Gay and Single . . . Forever?* Steven Bereznai mused, "I wonder if some of us simply get our comforting opiates from the Zen of solitude, free from the bustle of mindless chatter and the demands partners often seem to place on each other, robbing one of the possibility of immersing oneself in the pleasure of one's own company."[159] Quiet solitude can be especially appealing to the single at heart when we've already had our fill of socializing. "I can't do fragmented 'small talk,' and I find parties frustrating," David told me. "When in one of these situations, I can hardly wait to be happily home again, alone with my books, my artwork, my writings, my foods and comforts, and my own schedule."

We Get to Decide How to Use Our Space

When I wander bleary-eyed to the bathroom in the middle of the night, I never have to turn on the light to see if the seat was left up. If I put a soda in my fridge, then go to work—when I get home, it's still there! I am the queen of my remote control and my finances. The only underwear I wash are mine. I control the thermostat and the dinner menu.

I don't have to clear my schedule with anyone.

—Sonya (forty-seven, Parkersburg, West Virginia)

The single at heart love the autonomy and the independence we have when we are alone, the way we get to arrange our lives exactly as we please, even in the most mundane ways. For those of us who live alone, autonomy and independence also mean using our space however we like, conventions be damned.

Step into the living room of my home and the first thing you will notice is that my L-shaped desk dominates the room. The two tall bookcases have their say too. Sure, my living room has a comfy couch and chair, a coffee table and a TV, but really, it is my office and my study first of all.

I head to my desk the moment I wake up. Sometimes I bring my snacks there. From my desk, I can see the TV, so if there is something I want to vaguely monitor without leaving my work, I can do that too.

I didn't have to put my office in my living room. I have a guest bedroom I could have used. But the living room is my brightest, most spacious room, with views of lush greenery and even a peak of the Pacific Ocean. Whether I am working or just relaxing, it is where I want to be.

It is a bit offbeat, putting my office in my living room. It suggests an expansive view of what a living room is for. It is authentic too: I love my work. It is a big piece of what defines me. It deserves a place of prominence in my home as well as my life. I appreciate that I can make independent decisions about my space, without consulting anyone first. I'm unafraid of what people will think. All those qualities—authenticity, expansiveness, independence, being offbeat and unafraid of defying norms—are characteristic of people who are single at heart.

Really, though, my office example is only a little bit unconventional, and only one example of how people who are single at heart make their house a home that is truly their own. When I asked Kendra what made her happy, she said, "Being able to take up almost my entire living room to learn to paint." Kendra was divorced for the second time in her late twenties and raised her son on her own. Once her son was grown and she had her place to herself, she wasn't so sure at first that she would like living alone. Now she revels in the joy of it.

For Amy (forty-four, Frisco, Texas), her living room is for her dogs. She shared, "My younger dog is currently learning dog agility, so I have her agility weave poles set up in my living room. I literally moved the coffee table and brought her outdoor agility equipment inside! My living room looks nuts right now, but it works for me, and my dogs love being able to play with the agility equipment indoors (especially when it gets so hot outside)!"

Acadia, age thirty-six, loves music; her piano is in her bedroom. Her work desk is in the dining room.

David has been in broadcasting for nearly half a century. He's been a production manager for a TV station, a host for Austin's classical music station, and a local host for the Metropolitan Opera's live broadcasts. After decades of award-winning creative work, he started his own business producing programs and commercials. It is located in his living room. When David is inspired in the middle of the night, he gets up and goes to his workspace, where he blitzes on his creative projects for as long as his heart desires. He loves that. He was married previously. He knows that setting up shop in the living room or having odd and unpredictable hours is not always so straightforward with a spouse in the house.

Defanging the Horror Stories About Living Alone and Spending Time Alone

In the supreme importance that we place on intimate relationships, have we overlooked the deep, sustaining power of solitude in human life? [160]
—Anthony Storr

Storr posed that question in his classic 1988 work, *Solitude: A Return to the Self,* perhaps the most important book ever written on the topic. He believes that the capacity to be alone is a sign of emotional maturity. Yet in the decades that followed the book's publication, we have continued to be consumed with the supposedly supreme importance of intimate romantic relationships. We have feared, rather than celebrated, the place of solitude in our lives.

Living alone, spending time alone, social isolation, and loneliness have been tossed together into the same stew and served back to us in a cauldron of harrowing statistics. One of those statistics from a staid academic journal slipped the bonds of those musty pages and landed in the *New Yorker* in the form of this claim: "Social isolation is as deadly as smoking up to fifteen cigarettes a day."[161]

Some studies do in fact show that spending time alone is linked to anxiety, depression, loneliness, and a whole host of other maladies, and that social isolation can be deadly.[162] Another set of studies, though, show just how enriching it can be to spend time alone.[163] Solitude fosters creativity and spirituality. Free of the potentially distracting and judgmental presence of others, we can think more clearly, access our feelings more deeply, and ponder profound questions about who we are and who we want to be. Solitude is also a place of lightness and peace, of rest, restoration, and relaxation. Alone, we are free to do whatever it is we most enjoy.

A study of more than sixteen thousand people demolished the myth that people who live alone are lonelier.[164] When the solo dwellers were compared to people living with others who were similar to them in important ways, such as their economic security, the people who lived alone were *less* lonely.

So which is it? Is solitude harmful or beneficial? The latest research indicates that what matters is not just the amount of time people spend alone, but how that stacks up to the amount of alone time they want and need. Carleton University professor Robert J. Coplan and his colleagues have shown that people who do not get as much time to themselves as they would like report the same side effects as those who have too much unwanted time alone: they feel stressed, depressed, and unhappy with their lives.[165]

The most powerful factor separating risky solitude from psychologically fulfilling solitude is the "why" factor, the reasons people are alone. People who long to be included, for example, but who are instead forgotten, ostracized, or rejected, often find solitude devastating.[166] It is entirely different for the single at heart who love the time they have to themselves, who have chosen solitude, and who protect it like the precious resource it is to them. They are the ones who reap the rewards that all happy solitude-seekers enjoy.

People who are single at heart are not doomed to suffer the same fate as people who smoke fifteen cigarettes a day. Our love of solitude is not a vulnerability. It is one of our superpowers.

Flipping the Script

"In the past year that we've been under lockdown, I've cooked mainly just for myself . . . . I have enjoyed it immensely. In the same way, I feel I've been shown a troubling, relatively new tendency in myself to be alone for so long without being lonely." [167]
—Nigella Lawson

The ability to be alone without feeling lonely is a great skill, not something troubling. Imagine if she had instead said this: "In the past year that we've been under lockdown, I've cooked mainly for other people. I have enjoyed it immensely. In the same way, I feel I've been shown a troubling, relatively new tendency in myself to be with other people for so long without wishing I were single and living alone."

Advice For the Single at Heart

Recognize that your love of solitude is something rare and valuable. When so many other people are looking for reassurance that it is possible to be alone without feeling lonely, you already know that in your bones. When so many others are searching for guidance on how to enjoy spending time on their own, you don't need any instructions.

Be a teacher, a myth-buster, and an ambassador for solitude. Did you just have a busy week spending lots of time with other people? Don't hesitate to mention how much you are looking forward to having some time to yourself. Then, when asked about your weekend, offer the answer that hardly anyone expects: "It was glorious—I had it all to myself!"

Are you someone who loves their solitude but does not need a lot of it, even after a busy week? By unapologetically effusing about how much you savor both your solitude and your socializing, you can help people understand that it is perfectly natural to enjoy both.

For Our Allies

Understand that we like our alone time—it is not scary or lonely, it is fulfilling. Most of us enjoy socializing as well, so include us in your plans and accept our invitations to join us in our plans (and don't back out at the last minute!).

If you are a parent or a teacher or you have some other role in the lives of children, be sensitive to the natural and psychologically healthy differences among kids. Some children are contented spending time alone; they are not alone because they've been ostracized or bullied.[168] Allow children to spend time on their own instead of trying to schedule every moment; it will serve them well throughout their lives to feel comfortable when alone. Don't use isolation (such as a time-out) as punishment. Let children see you immersed in your reading, working on solo projects, or getting lost in your own thoughts.

If you are a therapist or other mental health professional, consider what Anneli Rufus said about you in *Party of One*, her book about people who like being alone: "If they ask whether we are alone by choice, they are doing their job. If they do not try to dissuade us, fine. If they move on from there to praise our self-awareness, our skill at choosing and living as we choose, they are doing their job. If they show us how to handle the slander, censure, jokes, and misapprehension . . . then they are doing their job."[169]

For Those Who Are Intrigued By Single Life, But Wonder Whether They Will Ever Be As Comfortable in Solitude as the Single at Heart

Remind yourself of the kinds of things you already enjoy doing on your own, such as exercising or shopping, or watching movies at home when no one else is around.

Plan to spend some extra time by yourself, a little at a time. You are especially likely to enjoy that alone time if you are doing something you are good at or something you find engaging. Don't use it to tackle the assignments or chores that you loathe.

Remember that when you are alone, you can also be meaningfully connected with other people, by thinking about them, emailing or texting them, or participating in online discussions.

Or forget about other people. Think of your alone time as freedom to do what you want to do and be who you want to be, with no concerns about what anyone else might think.

Don't force it! The moment you start thinking about spending time alone as something you *should* do, you have left the land of the single at heart.

The best advice for living fearlessly in solitude may also be the most challenging: figure out who you really are, then live your life accordingly. That way, when you are alone with yourself, you are with someone who is authentic.

5

The Ones

These women are the absolute foundation of my current life. Because
of them, I was comfortable buying a house by myself and putting down
roots somewhere. Because of them, I am inspired to build a life that is
truly what I want, not just what people expect. Because of them,
I am finally picking up my camera again after years of fear and
making something of that passion. Because of them,
I am happier now than I have ever been.
—Carla (thirty-three, Essex, England)

When I think about people who are great at friendship, I think about
Carla. I love how she and her friends have been there for one another
in ways that are big and small. I love how Carla acknowledges how much her
friends mean to her. I love that Carla shared her vulnerability with them, and
now with the readers of this book. I love how, with the help of those friends,
Carla's fear was transformed into strength, passion, and delight.

In Chapter 1, I described the joy, psychological richness, and
authenticity that are at the core of a single at heart life. Carla's friendships
contributed to all of those dimensions of her life. Because of her friends,
Carla is happier than she has ever been. She also has a psychologically rich
life because of them. She bought a house, picked up her camera, and followed
her passions. Having those friends in her life is itself a source of psychological
richness. Perhaps most significantly, Carla's friends championed her quest
for authenticity: "Because of them, I am inspired to build a life that is truly
what I want, not just what people expect."

People who do not understand what it means to flourish as a single
person do not expect stories like Carla's. They never questioned the prevailing

storyline that insists that if you want to have someone you can count on to be there for you, you need to find a romantic partner, prioritize that person, and build your life around that partner. Many feel secure in that conventional approach to life, rarely recognizing the riskiness of investing nearly all of their emotional and relationship capital into just one person. It might not even matter if they did understand their own vulnerability—it is the life they really want, just as my single life is the life I really want.

In the single at heart quiz, I asked, "Ideally who would be the most important adults in your life?" Of those who were clearly *not* single at heart, 88 percent gave the answer that, to them, must have seemed self-evident: they wanted a spouse or romantic partner to be the one most important adult in their life. But among those who clearly *were* single at heart, a nearly identical number, 89 percent, said that they did *not* want a romantic partner to be the one most important person in their life. They prefer other options.

Having a posse of friends, as Carla does, is one of those options. Many other people who are single at heart have a whole convoy of humans and nonhumans who have sailed with them through their lives, including, for example, relatives, mentors, spiritual figures, pets, and maybe even casual romantic partners, as well as friends. Some of the single at heart have people in their lives who are not family in the usual sense of the term, but who are so much like family in all the best ways that they think of them as their chosen families. Others do not organize their lives around other people at all, and that works too.

Our Friends

In opposition to the accepted order of things, for many of us, it's our friendships that need to be at the top of our love hierarchy if we want to live long and happy lives. Friends can be our sources of intimacy and nonjudgmental support, they can be our life's companions, they can be our family and our co-parent. Put bluntly, they're our survival.[170]

—Anna Machin, "Treasure Them"

After decades of obsessive preoccupation with the study of marriage and romantic partnerships, scholars are increasingly turning their attention to friends. What they are finding must be making them wonder what took them so long. In an extraordinary survey of more than three hundred thousand adults, including representative national samples from ninety-nine nations, Peiqi Lu of Columbia University and her colleagues found that friendship was important all around the world.[171] The people who said that friends had a more important place in their lives were generally happier, healthier, and more satisfied with their lives.

The special place of friends in our lives is evident from studies that average across all people, regardless of their marital or relationship status, as the ninety-nine-nation study did. When single people are compared to married or coupled people, it is the single people who are more likely to have more friends, to hold onto their friends, and to experience even greater joy from spending time with them.[172] For the people who are not just single, but single at heart, our investment in our friends, and the rewards we reap from having them in our lives, are often greater still.

It's not that I loved my friends any less, but I couldn't maintain
that level of daily commitment to them if I was also going
to make room for my boyfriend.[173]
—Rebecca Traister, author of *All the Single Ladies: Unmarried
Women and the Rise of an Independent Nation*

When she said that about her friends, Traister was explaining to best-selling author Roxane Gay how prioritizing her boyfriend and then marrying him had changed her. People who are single at heart don't do that. We do not aspire to put a romantic partner at the center of our lives, so we are unlikely to demote our friends to accommodate such a partner.

The sociologists Naomi Gerstel and Natalia Sarkisian have conducted a program of research on what they call "greedy marriage," which is the way in which married couples invest most of their time and attention in each other, and marginalize other people such as friends, neighbors, siblings, and parents.[174] Using data from two nationally representative surveys of adults in the US, they compared the efforts made by lifelong single people, previously married people, and married people to maintain their ties with the people in their lives. In every comparison, the single people did more than anyone else. Married people usually did the least, with the previously married in between. For example, the single people were most likely to socialize with their neighbors and their friends at least several times a month. They were most likely to see their parents at least once a week. They ranked first in giving friends, neighbors, coworkers, siblings, and parents "advice, encouragement, and moral or emotional support; help with shopping, errands, or transportation; help with housework, yard work, car repairs, or other work around the house; or help with child care," and receiving comparable help from them.[175]

The results were the same for the men as for the women, for the rich and the poor, and for blacks, whites, and Hispanics: The lifelong single people did the most to nurture their social ties. Gerstel and Sarkisian tried to determine whether factors other than marital status could explain the results, but none of them did.[176] For example, the single people's greater efforts to maintain their various relationships could not be explained by being at a different point in their life course, working fewer hours, or not having kids. (Even couples who do not have kids do less to maintain their social ties than single people do.)

In *Friends: Understanding the Power of Our Most Important Relationships*, the acclaimed British evolutionary psychologist Robin Dunbar reports that "falling in love will cost you two friendships."[177] People who follow a conventional life path—being single and not dating, then dating, then cohabiting or marrying, then having kids, and then becoming empty nesters—seem to shed or marginalize their friends all along the way.

The Dutch professor of Demography Matthijs Kalmijn documented that pattern when he compared people who were in each of those categories.[178] The people who were single and not dating were in touch with their close friends an average of thirteen or fourteen times a month; the people who were empty nesters were in contact only five or six times a month. The biggest drop in attending to friends was between the single people who were not dating and those who were. For the men, especially, there was another big drop between the singles who were dating and those who moved in with a partner or married them.

In the US, Kelly Musick and Larry Bumpass zeroed in on that second drop. They followed more than twenty-seven hundred people for years, starting when they were under fifty and not married or cohabiting. They found that the people who got married or moved in with a romantic partner became more insular.[179] They spent less time with their friends than they had when they were single. They were in touch with their parents less often too. It wasn't just a matter of temporary infatuation. Six years later, they were still spending less time with their friends and contacting their parents less often than they had been when they were single.

When I was little, one of my favorite people was the boy next door. We spent many long summer days with the other neighborhood kids, playing baseball until it got so dark we could barely see. When we were teens, we switched to tennis.

He was never my boyfriend. We were friends. My whole life, I have had important platonic friends who are men. I never experienced male friendship as overlaid with any weird interpersonal dynamics. That popular question, "Can men and women really be 'just friends'?" seemed baffling. Why shouldn't they be?

Other people who are single at heart seem to feel similarly. For example, Sonya (forty-seven, Parkersburg, West Virginia) said, "I have friends of all genders." Joan (seventy-three, Newark, Delaware) has had platonic, emotionally intimate relationships with about a dozen men. As she shared, "The fact that they were men was largely irrelevant, because they accept the fact that I don't want a romantic relationship and value my friendship on its own terms."

While people who are pursuing long-term romantic coupling are sidelining their friends, people who are single at heart are continuing their lifelong practice of opening their arms to all sorts of potential friends. We are particularly expansive in our friendships *because* we are single at heart. If deep down you just aren't all that interested in long-term romantic coupling, then the world does not sort itself into potential romantic partners and potential platonic friends. Everyone is a potential friend, and their gender, gender identity, or sexual orientation simply doesn't matter.

> I marvel at the support I've derived from friends.
> In their constant embrace, I have never felt alone.[180]
> —Sonia Sotomayor, US Supreme Court Justice

The people who unsingle themselves and then marginalize their friends are losing out on many of the gifts of friendship. They are missing out on the delight of being with friends and the protection from loneliness and depression that friendship offers. They don't enjoy the same boosts to their self-esteem. They may not find their lives as fulfilling. They may also be forsaking some of the best opportunities to be who they really are.

When Nobel Prize winner Daniel Kahneman and his colleagues asked 909 women to report who they were with the day before and how they felt during each of their social interactions, they found that the women were happiest when they were with their friends.[181] Spending time with other kinds of people, such as spouses, romantic partners, relatives, children, or coworkers, just didn't seem to be as emotionally rewarding.

In early adulthood, people without romantic partners are already moving toward their friends while people with partners are moving away from them. That's what social psychologist Alexandra N. Fisher and her colleagues found when they studied 279 students over the course of two years of college, checking in with them eight times.[182] Over time the students who did not have a romantic partner felt closer and closer to their friends, and any doubts about those friendships began to dissipate. They had invested in their friends. By doing so, they had also invested in themselves: the better they felt about their friendships, the better they felt about themselves. It was different for the students with romantic partners; on average, the quality of their friendships declined. They were not reaping the boosts to their self-esteem that their unpartnered peers were enjoying. Meanwhile, on average, the quality of their romantic relationship was not improving either.

In his analyses of survey data from more than 250 thousand adults older than thirty in thirty-two European nations, Hebrew University sociologist Elyakim Kislev found that for people of all marital statuses, spending more time socializing with friends (and relatives and colleagues) was linked to greater happiness.[183] The people without romantic partners, though, socialized more than the cohabiting or married people did. They were doing more of just the sort of thing, socializing, that filled everyone's life with happiness. What's more, the link between socializing and happiness was stronger for them. The single people got even more joy out of the time they spent with their friends.

Single people who want to be single put more into their friendships and get more out of them than single people who want to be coupled. Over the course of a nine-year study of nearly six thousand German divorced and lifelong single people, Kislev found that wanting to be single and valuing friends were intertwined in a virtuous circle.[184] The more those adults wanted to be single, the more they valued their friendships. In turn, as they found their friendships more fulfilling, they found their single lives more fulfilling too. Meanwhile, those who were pining for a partner were growing more disillusioned by their friendships. They valued them less, invested in them less, and then they yearned even more for that one special romantic relationship.

Anna Machin, who made the case earlier in this chapter for why friendships may belong at the very top of our love hierarchies, also believes that friendships beautifully honor the authenticity that the single at heart value so highly: "My work has shown that our friendships can provide a level of understanding and emotional intimacy that can eclipse any we might experience with a lover. Indeed, friends are often the most reliable source of an interpersonal ease, allowing us to be our true selves."

She was talking about all people, not just the single at heart, noting that just about everyone feels more authentic when they are with their friends. The single at heart do have an advantage though. We don't think of any of our friends as potential long-term romantic partners, so we aren't trying to present a version of ourselves that might transform a friend into a romantic partner. We love our friends just the way they are, as friends. When we are with them, we can be just the way we are, our true selves.[185]

The people we interviewed were consciously seeking to create a way of life that would meet their need for connection with others while preserving their autonomy and independence. They placed a high value on the way in which friends offer care and support, love and affection without infringing personal boundaries . . . . [They valued] both attachments to others and self-determination.[186]
—Sasha Roseneil, "Why We Should Care About Friends"

The people Professor Roseneil had interviewed, along with her colleague Shelley Budgeon, were a diverse group of fifty-three people in the UK, ages twenty-five through sixty, who did not live with a romantic partner. Some had children and some had romantic partners they weren't living with, but "very few showed any yearning to be part of a conventional couple or family."[187] They loved and valued their friends, and their commitment to them was profound. "It was friends far more than biological kin who offered support to those who suffered from emotional distress or mental health problems," Roseneil reported. "Friends were invited to stay during periods of homelessness, when out of work, or when they were depressed or lonely."[188] Some had even moved or persuaded their friends to move, so they could be near one another in case of illness or to help with childcare for those who had kids—as well as to enjoy their company in the good times and the bad.

Eighteen months after they first interviewed those fifty-three people, Roseneil and Budgeon contacted them again and found that they were still prioritizing their friends. "This was not a temporary phase and people did not return to conventional couple relationships as soon as an opportunity arose."[189]

For the single at heart, friends are wonderful people to have in our lives. In our quest to lead joyful, psychologically rich, and authentic lives, lives full of freedom and autonomy balanced with just the right amount of companionship and closeness, no other kind of relationship partner is likely to be as superb as a friend. We cherish the companionship, warmth, and care that we and our friends provide one another, and we especially appreciate that we can feel connected and supported without losing the freedom and autonomy that are so dear to us.

Friendships don't come burdened with the gendered roles and expectations that can plague even the most progressive of heterosexual romantic relationships. Friendships are not freighted with the normative expectations and obligations of other relationships, such as family ties. We may well help our parents and other relatives even more often than coupled people do, as research suggests, but we prefer to help because we want to and not because it is what we "should" do.

We don't aspire to become enmeshed in another person's life, the way some couples do. We prefer the space that friendships offer us to stand back and guiltlessly savor our solitude when we want to, or to socialize with as many different people as we like, of any gender, as often as we like. Friends are less likely to feel threatened by that than a romantic partner might. They are not going to sit us down and insist on having the talk about where the relationship is going.

Our friendships can hit rough patches and even implode spectacularly, leaving us feeling devastated, just as anyone's can. But the death of our friendships is not going to come at the hands of a jealous romantic partner, or at least not *our* jealous romantic partner.

Our Chosen Families

What I love about found family is that it can accommodate
all the love and meals and holidays and hospital visits of any other
family—all the true confessions and late-night conversations
and child chaos and quotidian mess and hugs and
endearments and quantity time; and yet it is often kinder
than original family, and more miraculous, because it is a
gift given when you are old enough to appreciate it,
a commitment continuously made when you know what
that commitment costs and means. A family found in
adulthood can never attain the involuntary intimacy of the siblings
who have known you since birth, and squabbled with you in
bathrooms and at breakfast tables from time immemorial.
But sometimes, perhaps for this reason, a found family can
know and love you for who you are—not for who you once were,
or who you never were.[191]

—Briallen Hopper, *Hard to Love*

People who fill conventional family roles, such as brothers and sisters, husbands and wives, and parents and children, are expected to have special places in our lives and in our hearts. That's the sentimentalized version of family. Sometimes, though, the families we choose as adults, that include people who are not related to us by blood, adoption, or marriage, are among the people we love and cherish more than anyone else. Hopper calls them "found families," but there are other terms as well, such as "families of choice," "logical families," and my least favorite, "fictive kin" (sounds like the people are make believe).

Chosen family members can foster the joy, psychological richness, and authenticity that are so significant to the single at heart. Hopper was documenting the joy of found family when she pointed to the love, hugs, endearments, quality time, and kindness. There is a psychological richness, a mindfulness, in what she described as "a commitment continuously made," the process of choosing over and over again to be there for one another, when neither law nor custom demands it. And perhaps most importantly, Hopper explains how found families honor authenticity; they "know and love you for who you are—not for who you once were, or who you never were."

When we choose our families, we are often choosing friends, but just about anyone in any role can be included. When Sonya (forty-seven, Parkersburg, West Virginia) told me about her chosen family, she began by talking about friends and then included children too:

> My best friend of over thirty years and her husband are my chosen family. We have helped each other with moving, household tasks requiring more than one person, financially, going to medical appointments, etc. We are each other's emergency contact. Her husband is my MPOA [medical power of attorney]. We also take vacations together, spend holidays together, and get together socially often. My best friend and I work together, and chat outside of work hours every day. As godmother to her three children, I played the "surrogate soccer mom" for several years as they grew up. When all three had events going on at the same time, they knew either Mom, Dad, or Aunt Sonya would be there cheering them on. Now that the kids are grown, they still come to see me, attend social events at my house, etc. In every way except blood, we are family.

Carla is an only child, but she has three "sisters of choice." They are the friends who would drop everything to be there for her in a crisis, as she would for them. Her mother considers them "extra daughters." Liz (sixty, Washington, DC) said, "I consider myself a member of two families—one is of blood relatives and relatives by marriage consisting of my siblings, their spouses, their kids, my cousins etc., and another equally important one that consists of really good friends who are like family to me." Carmela (44, Nayarit, Mexico) has close friends from five families who live near her. Those families, she said, "adopted" her. She spends weekends and holidays with them.

> Sooner or later . . . no matter where in the world we live, we must join the diaspora, venturing beyond our biological family to find our logical one, the one that actually makes sense for us.[192]
> —Armistead Maupin, *Logical Family: A Memoir*

In choosing the people who matter most to them, rather than defaulting to a conventional romantic partner or nuclear family, people who are single at heart are continuing a tradition that other groups have created and championed. In anthropologist Kath Weston's award-winning 1991 book, *Families We Choose: Lesbians, Gays, Kinship*, she showed how people in queer communities in the US established families of their own.[193] Homophobia was more rampant in the nineties, and many lesbians and gays were motivated to create their own families because they were rejected by their families of origin. But even today, many members of sexual or gender minorities, including those who are fully accepted and even embraced by their original families, find value in creating and maintaining their own versions of family as well. Other queer people in particular can provide a kind of support and affirmation that original families often cannot.

In her overview of historical and contemporary notions of African American kinship, University of Georgia professor Chalandra M. Bryant pointed out that enslaved children were encouraged to refer to unrelated adults as "aunt" and "uncle."[194] That practice fostered close bonds and created vital networks of support. The continued significance of chosen family is evident today in a rich vocabulary of terms of affection and inclusion. For example, groups of black male friends with especially strong bonds of loyalty are referred to as "going for brothers." "Othermothers" are women who help to care for children who are not their own and who support the mothers of those children too. "Play brothers" or "play sisters" start off as friends and then become more like family—they are "playing at" being a brother or sister. "Sister circles," which are networks of friends, have been important to African American women for 150 years, Bryant notes.

In her 2020 study of single black women, Wayne State University scholar Jessica D. Moorman found that many had robust social networks that sometimes included relatives and previous romantic partners as well as friends.[195] When these women needed rides, a hand with chores or childcare, financial assistance, or support when they were ill or facing a crisis, both their conventional family and their chosen family were often there for them.

Asked whether they had someone to whom they were not related, but who they treated just like a relative, nine out of ten adults in a nationally representative sample of African Americans, black Caribbeans, and non-Hispanic whites said that they did.[196] The African Americans and black Caribbeans had even more people in that category than the whites did. They were also especially likely to feel close to people in their churches or other places of worship; those people too can be honored as chosen family.

The strength of friendship networks—and their ability to promote community—rests on their separateness from family and cohabitation.[197]
—E. Kay Trimberger, *The New Single Woman*

For centuries, people have been using the language of family to describe the important people in their lives who are not family in any conventional sense. Calling someone a sister or brother, an auntie or uncle, suggests a certain warmth and closeness that is not so routinely associated with friends, who are too often referred to as "just friends." "Family" implies security: they will be there for you. That's their role. "Family" also confers legitimacy. It is family, not friendship, that is protected by laws in countries such as the US and recognized and valued in our everyday lives.

Professor E. Kay Trimberger wants this to stop. When we lovingly describe our friends as family, we are highlighting the sentimentalized notion of family and obscuring the ways in which families can inflict pain, cause harm, and perpetuate inequality. No one ever says, "He's just like family to me. He abused me over and over again." We are pretending that a spouse or family member really can be counted on to be there when needed, always and forever, and that there is no such thing as estrangement from family. We are propping up the Magical Mythical Romantic Partner.

When we use the language of family to describe our friends, Trimberger believes, we are unwittingly contributing to the devaluing of friends by masking their significance. Our networks of friends are often less insular than conventional families and therefore can connect us to our communities more nimbly. Often it is our friends who show up for us when we are in need; we honor what they have done for us when we call them friends rather than sisters, even though family terms are intended as high compliments and special expressions of love.

Trimberger also recognizes that with friends, we can have companionship and love, and our freedom and autonomy too. That's especially so when we don't live with them. She pointed out that the communes that became popular in the US in the 1960s and 1970s rarely lasted longer than a few years. The people who joined those communes were often white middle-class youth who longed for an alternative to the nuclear families they grew up in. What they didn't realize is that the togetherness they craved was not so wonderful when it wasn't balanced with privacy, freedom, and autonomy.

For the single at heart, freedom and autonomy are essential. Sonya said that her best friend, her best friend's husband, and their three kids were family "in every way except blood." Sonya, though, had a place of her own.

I've mentioned Carla's friends before, including the three she described as sisters. She has other cherished humans and nonhumans in her life too.

Importantly, she also has her freedom. "I have commitments: my mom and gran, lots of friends and family and my cats," she said, "but I have freedom to organize my life in the way that I want to."

None of this means that people who are single at heart cannot live with other people amicably and lovingly. Some do. Twenty-six-year-old Yogesh, for example, lives with his parents in Karnal, India. Andrea (29, New York City), Yolanda (26, Washington, DC), and Alyssa (27, Los Angeles) have roommates. People who are coupled, but who insist that "at heart" they are really single, sometimes share a place with a romantic partner. And, of course, some people who are single at heart are raising kids. Typically, though, it is more of a challenge for the single at heart to live the joyful, psychologically rich, and authentic lives that they love when they don't have a place of their own.

Our Convoys of Humans and Nonhumans

I am always in relationship to my ancestors or my spirit guides.
I am in relationship to the sun. I am in relationship to my family
members and friends and my pets and my plants.
And so I'm never really alone in this world.[198]
—Jayda Shuavarnnasri, "Asian Auntie," APEX radio

To be single at heart is to have an openhearted approach to relationships. To us the word "relationship" isn't shorthand for a romantic relationship. We can have relationships with all sorts of humans and nonhumans.

For decades, University of Michigan professor Toni C. Antonucci and her colleagues have been studying "social convoys," the people who accompany us over the course of our lives.[199] Unlike many other scholars, Professor Antonucci has never presumed that certain categories of people would be more important than others. Instead, in true single at heart spirit, she invites the people she studies to tell her about the people in their lives. She asks who is in their inner circle ("people to whom you feel so close that it is hard to imagine life without them"), their middle circle (not quite as close as the inner circle, but still important), and their outer circle (not as close as the people in the other circles, but still a part of your personal network).

Our social convoys can include anyone at all—friends, parents, siblings, children, other relatives, in-laws, romantic partners and ex-partners, neighbors, mentors, professional helpers, teammates, and coworkers, among others. The people who are not included can be just as telling as those who are; for example, married people do not always include their spouse. The makeup of our social convoy changes over the course of our lives, as some people die or move away, geographically or emotionally, and others become newly important to us. Typically, though, there is some stability as well.

The participants in the research on social convoys are asked about the people in their lives, but they don't always limit themselves to naming humans or living humans. Similarly, when people who are single at heart tell me about who matters to them, some of them name entities such as pets, spiritual figures, and deceased friends, relatives, and pets, as well as living humans. When "Asian Auntie" Jayda Shuavarnnasri said that she was in relation to ancestors, spirit guides, family, friends, pets, plants, and the sun, she was describing what she had learned from Indigenous traditions, as described, for example, by professor of Native Studies Kim TallBear.[200] The most inclusive, expansive, openhearted perspectives on relationships are the ones most likely to resonate with people who are single at heart.

Although he was single, he had a community of people he liked.[201]
—Vivek H. Murthy, MD, *Together*
Fixed it!
Like so many other single people, he had a community of people he liked.

Isn't It Easier to Have "The One" Than "The Ones"?

A journalist who interviewed me said that she had talked to a lot of single people and they all effused about their friends. She was skeptical. She had a boyfriend—"The One" rather than "The Ones"—and she thought that worked out better. If she wanted to go out to dinner, a movie, or a football game, she had someone to go with her. Wasn't it different for me? When I wanted to do fun things, wouldn't I have to figure out who was available, if anyone, then plan the event from scratch each time? Wasn't that kind of tiresome?

In the twenty years I lived in Charlottesville, Virginia, I had regular social events that required little or no planning. On weekdays I had lunch with colleagues. A few times a week I met friends for dinner on the downtown mall. On Sundays I often hosted an evening of watching bad TV at my place. I was also part of a cooking club that met every couple of months for ten years. A few years after moving to Summerland, California, I met a man at a writers conference who was the one other person out of hundreds who was interested in social science writing. We have had dinner about once month ever since—eighteen years and counting.

Even if I did not have regularly scheduled social events, I would not want what the journalist wanted. Overwhelmingly, other people who are single at heart don't either. One of the single at heart quiz items asked, "Many couples expect to be each other's 'plus-one' for just about every occasion. How do you feel about that?" Of the single at heart, 94 percent said they would prefer more options. Of the people who were not single at heart, 68 percent said they took comfort in having a person in their life to be their plus-one.

Many of us like the psychological richness of socializing with a variety of people. We like the flexibility and the freedom of doing what we want, including not going to that party at all and just staying home. I think we are also less fazed by the prospect of doing things in public on our own. I've waltzed into many social events dominated by couples, and rather than feeling self-conscious, I feel proud. I didn't succumb to the pressure to couple up in order to have an easier time at those kinds of events, and I don't slink out early or not show up at all out of embarrassment. Sometimes I wonder how many of the other people at the event are coupled not because they are enjoying a profoundly fulfilling relationship, but because they are afraid to be single.

• • • •

As a single, I have none of the traditional boundaries, which means I have
friends of all kinds. All my friends have their own specialties. If I have
a spiritual need, I have a handful of friends that I would turn to. These
may not be the same friends I would turn to with an intellectual need
or an emotional need. Singles are more likely to turn to someone who
can actually assist rather than depend on a monogamous partner for
assistance in an area that may not be their strength—
and then resent them for not having an ability.
—Sonya (forty-seven, Parkersburg, West Virginia)

I don't have nearly as many people in my personal network as some others who are single at heart do. But I do have someone I turn to when I have good news. I know she is going to be excited for me, in an uncomplicated way. I have a different person I seek out when I'm distraught about something. I know I can count on her. When I'm brimming with righteous anger, though, I want to vent with the person who is most likely to share my outrage, and that's usually someone else entirely.

That's not very efficient of me to seek out different people for different emotional needs. If I had a long-term romantic partner, I could just slip my feelings into the ongoing conversation of our lives. Wouldn't that be better? Research shows that it's not. A trio of social scientists compared people with a diverse portfolio of what they call "emotionships" to people who mostly share with the same person regardless of how they are feeling. They found that the people with The Ones tended to be more satisfied with their lives.[202]

I think Marie (forty-six, Northern California) was describing emotionships when she said, "I am closest to my sister, but have an intentional small circle of eclectic friends. They allow me to explore my many layers." Liz (sixty, Washington, DC) has different friends for different interests: "There is the gay man with whom I go on road trips, the friend who I go to see movies with, the theater buff who is my companion when I wish to see plays, the foodies who like trying out new restaurants like I do, and the potluck and other dinners I have with friends." Having a variety of interesting and unique experiences is one of the hallmarks of a psychologically rich life, and people who have The Ones rather than The One are more likely to have those kinds of experiences.

> I don't have anyone to share the burden if the water heater breaks,
> or the car won't start, or there's a dead mouse in the garage;
> nor do I have to check with them on what they
> think about the water heater, or the car, or the mouse.
> —Joan (seventy-three, Newark, Delaware)

There are many times when I wish I had another person around to help with the chores and those random things that go wrong. But in the trade-off Joan describes between having someone to help and having to take that person's preferences into account, the single at heart tilt toward wanting to do things our own way. We like being the deciders. Also, for many of us, our love of living alone trumps all else. I don't want someone to help with the dishes or the car if that means I have to live with someone.

Surveys that ask single people if they want to marry consistently find that the answer depends on whether the single person has ever been married.[203] People who have never been married are much more likely to say they want to marry than people who are divorced or widowed. Maybe that's in part because the previously married aren't so wowed by the Magical Mythical Romantic Partner. They know that the dream of having a partner who shares equally and happily with household tasks can turn out to be nothing more than a fantasy. For couples, the division of labor is such an emotionally charged issue that social scientists have published many thousands of articles, books, and dissertations trying to understand it. That hasn't helped much. Unequal burdens (and battles over them) continue to be part of coupled life.

When my outpatient minor surgery is scheduled, I need to prove that I've
got sufficient connections to get myself a ride home. As a single self-
employed person, newly relocated, with no relatives living nearby with
time on their hands, this requirement becomes more stressful than the
surgery itself. Why should I be denied care if I'm single and
new in town? For that matter, why must I be a friendly,
sociable person who attracts dozens of caring friends?
Can't I be a curmudgeonly hermit and still get medical care?[204]
—Cathy Goodwin, "How Hospitals Do Us Wrong

That journalist I mentioned previously who asked me skeptical
questions about the value of friends wondered about something else too.
She had had a medical appointment recently and needed a ride home. That
was no problem; of course, her boyfriend would drive her. Isn't that more of
a hassle for single people?

It can be. It is an issue that comes up repeatedly in my conversations
with single people, and not just the single at heart. For some medical
outpatient procedures in the US, patients are required to have someone
to drive them, and taxi or Uber drivers are not allowed. The problem is
compounded when the precise time of the procedure is not set until the last
minute, so the person needing the ride has to ask someone to block off an
entire day for them.

Many people who are single at heart have friends who would help, but
as Cathy Goodwin noted, we should not have to have friends in order to
receive medical care. Plus, our friends have lives. We may not want to ask
them to take a day off from work or other commitments. And what if we are
just not ready to share the reason for needing a particular medical procedure,
not even with a friend?

The issue is not one that burdens only single people. Romantic partners
have lives too, often including jobs. For many coupled people, especially older
ones, their spouse or partner may not have the capacity to help, however willing

they may be. This is a structural problem, not a single's problem. Hospitals and other health care facilities that require patients to have rides should have a free or affordable transportation service available to all.

Do the Single at Heart Have Our Own Version of "The One"?

I believe in soul mates but I don't believe that you have to have sex with your soul mate or marry your soul mate. . . . I have four soul mates now. They are people for whom I would give my life. But I wouldn't have them come live with me in my house. I don't want to marry them. They are married to other people anyway.[205]
—Whoopi Goldberg, *If Someone Says, "You Complete Me," RUN!*

"What if friendship, not marriage, was at the center of life?", asked Rhaina Cohen in a 2020 article in *The Atlantic*.[206] Cohen profiled pairs of friends—"platonic partners"—whose lives were about as interconnected as any married couple's, except for the sex. For example, platonic partners might "live in houses they purchased together, raise each other's children, use joint credit cards, and hold medical and legal powers of attorney for each other."[207] The idea of prioritizing a friend rather than a romantic partner resonated far and wide. Cohen's article was wildly popular. On TikTok around the same time, videos about platonic life partners were attracting millions of views.

None of the single at heart who shared their life stories with me had a platonic life partner. It is likely that some people who are single at heart do have such partners and I just haven't heard from them, or they will in the future. Platonic partners offer more of the freedom that the single at heart cherish than romantic partners do. Platonic partners do not expect to be each other's one and only important friend. Loving another friend wouldn't be cheating. Platonic friends are also typically the same gender, and so they do not drift into the conventional gender roles characteristic of many heterosexual romantic couples, roles that are not very appealing to the single at heart.

Generally I think the single at heart are more likely to have The Ones than The One, even if The One is a platonic partner rather than a romantic one. Carla, for example, has three "sisters of choice," not one. And Whoopi Goldberg has four soulmates, not one. Like many people who are single at heart, Goldberg does not want to live with any of those people, even though she would give her life for them. Carla lives alone too. We who are single at heart need and love our solitude, and that's harder to come by if we build a life around a platonic partner. We can still have many people in our lives who we love and cherish without turning any of them into The One.

Flipping the Script

"For a significant number of people ... their friends fulfill the role of a romantic partner."[208]
—Anna Machin, "Treasure Them"

Professor Machin, who has written so compellingly about the power of friendship, still seems to be positioning a romantic partner as the key relationship everyone is expected to have; if they don't have it, friends can substitute. But friends should not be regarded as replacements. They are significant in and of themselves. Imagine if she had instead said: "For a significant number of people, their romantic partner fulfills the role of their friends."

When Other People Just Aren't That Important

I am my family. I trust me. I always have my back.
—Claudia (sixty-nine, Washington, DC)

I've said that people who are single at heart are more likely to have The Ones than The One, and made the case that having The Ones can be advantageous. Some people who are single at heart do not have The Ones or The One. Other people just don't have a particularly important role in their lives.

Claudia, who said "I am my family," is one example. Another is Ginny (fifty-nine, Ontario, Canada) who said that she was "interested in just about every aspect of the natural world but the lives of people just don't interest me." Acadia (thirty-six, Melbourne, Australia) used to experience feelings of dread when she was heading out to see her friends, even though she liked them. For her, the pandemic was transformative:

> For the first time in my life, the anxiety has left me. I feel completely calm and at peace, knowing there is no one to meet, no one to interact with, no obligation to put on my "outside" face and pretend I am enjoying myself.
>
> 2020 has made me more confident than ever that a solitary life is for me. I hope that when the pandemic is over, people respect those who have found solace in solitude and continue to allow them to have space to be themselves.

In a way, I feel more protective of these single at heart people than any of the others. I suspect they are most likely to be stigmatized by those who cannot understand how someone can say "I am my family" and still be healthy and happy. Some social scientists are skeptical too. Over and over again, socializing with other people has been linked to better health and a longer life.[209] I don't doubt the truth of those findings as a general principle. But when you read about the results of a study, you are hearing about the combined results, averaged across all the people who participated in the research. There are always people who stand apart from the trends, who, for example, are doing just fine even though they socialize far less than most people do, or do not look to any one person or network of persons they trust, to be there for them when they are in need.

The key question is whether the kind of life these people have chosen is working for them. For the people who are single at heart, it is. No single at heart person I've spoken with is unhappy with their life. While, like anyone, they may be unhappy with certain challenging areas of life (such as financial difficulties or health issues), they revel in the power, freedom, and heart-filling joy of single life. The single at heart flourish in their solitude, they do not feel lonely, and they are curious, with psychologically rich lives of the mind. Ginny, for example, is someone who *can* be social, the life of the party even, but only for a while. In contrast, there is no time limit on her capacity to be enthralled by the natural world.

Some, such as Acadia, tried and tried to be the kind of sociable person that just about everyone is expected to be, the kind of person who is most readily admired and understood. The pandemic gifted her with the opportunity to instead live the way she always felt most comfortable, and the courage to stand by her life of solitude even after the worst of COVID subsided.

Acadia is also deeply religious. She used to attend church in person, but during the pandemic, that was no longer possible. "I feel much closer to God now," she said, "as I am able to fully concentrate on His Word without feeling nervous about all the people around me and losing my focus." In experiencing profound spirituality while in solitude, Acadia is part of a long tradition that transcends any one religion or spiritual practice. In those traditions, alone time and quiet time are revered, not feared.

None of these people are at a loss when faced with challenges. They have their own ways of coping when things get tough. "I rely on a community of experts, business associates, friends, and acquaintances to help me through these things," Claudia said. "I also read a lot about the issue at hand, and plan for any potential difficulties. If things look like they might get out of hand, I call on a professional for help."

Social scientists are starting to look a bit more closely at the claims that more socializing is always better for you. They are finding instead that sometimes a little socializing goes a long way. A study of nearly four hundred thousand people from thirty-seven European nations showed that people who socialized several times a month did have better health than those who socialized less often, but there were hardly any additional health benefits to socializing more than a few times a month.[210] The findings were even more remarkable from a study in which close to fifty thousand Germans were surveyed for years. Again, seeing people about once a month was better than seeing people less often. But socializing with relatives more often than that was actually associated with worse health. And the people who socialized more than once a month—whether with relatives, friends, neighbors, or colleagues—did not live as long as the less sociable people.[211]

As always, the findings are based on averages across all the people in the study, and there are always exceptions. Some people can socialize constantly, including with relatives, and do just fine. The research, though, does caution us to think more carefully about what it could mean to spend a lot of time with other people. Sometimes our interactions with other people are stressful rather than comforting. And even if we enjoy every moment of our time with other people, that's time that we cannot devote to other pursuits we may also value, including just having more time to ourselves.

We Can Be Our Own Source of Comfort and Security

In 1991, my father died in what seemed like an instant. He had an aneurysm, it burst, and that was the end of that. He was just sixty-four. I was in Virginia and my parents lived hundreds of miles away in Pennsylvania. Before my mother called to tell me, she called one of my friends so that I could have someone to be with me if I wanted.

I didn't want it. It was the most stunning and devastating news I had ever received, but I did not want to turn to anyone else for comfort—not at first. I wanted to start processing it myself. Later, I would very much want to tell the story to people who cared about me.

I feel that way about other difficult news too, and even about extremely good news. I want to mull over the bad stuff or savor the good stuff, then look to the important people in my life.

I always thought that was just another way in which I wasn't like other people. Then in 2011 I was asked to serve as an outside member of Carol Kahn's dissertation committee at Drexel University. Kahn posed a radical question about attachment: Could single people be their own source of comfort and security? She conducted in-depth interviews with fourteen people, ranging in age from their late forties to their late eighties, who had always been single, had no children, and had not been in a committed romantic relationship for at least the previous five years.[212]

One of the questions Kahn asked was, "If you got really good news or really bad news right now, what would you do?" Eight of the fourteen people said that the first thing they would want to do would be to sit with the news on their own. Then, like me, they wanted to turn to others. Rather than having just one attachment figure, the single people Kahn studied had an attachment community. They had The Ones, not just The One.

Kahn found that the lifelong single people she interviewed seemed to have gotten to know themselves in particularly deep ways. She saw that self-knowledge not as an alternative to turning to other people, but an enhancement of it:

> The attachment community is made fuller and more mean-
> ingful by the interdependence of turning inward for self-
> care and connection to self with turning outward for con-
> nection to others.
>
> When something deeply significant happens, these single
> people first wanted to be with just one person—themselves.
> Then they turned to their community, The Ones they can
> count on, and who in turn, can count on them.

Advice for the Single at Heart

If friends are at the center of your life, you already take them seriously. Let other people know that. Mention your friends in conversations as readily as coupled people mention their partners. Talk about the meals you've shared, the outings you've enjoyed together, how you celebrated their birthdays, and how they were there for you when you really needed them. Show off photos of you with your friends so others remember their faces and see the kinds of experiences you share together.

Do the same for all the other kinds of humans who matter to you—and nonhumans too. Relatives, colleagues, and mentors are among the people who are important to some of us. Ancestors and spiritual figures can be significant as well. Pets too. Own your love of them.

If other people do not have a particularly important place in your life and that's how you like it, own that too. Over the centuries, many people have enjoyed meaningful and fulfilling lives focused on spirituality or work or passions or other pursuits in which other people did not figure prominently. You can be proud of your place in that tradition.

For Our Allies

Be a good friend to the single people in your lives. Show up for their birthdays and other important occasions. Ask your single friends and relatives about their friends—and their pets, if they have any. Let them know that a friend is just as welcome to be a plus-one as a romantic partner. Recognize that friend breakups can be painful and offer the same sympathy and comfort that you would to a person whose romantic relationship had ended. Understand that the deaths of close friends and relatives—and pets—can be devastating. If you are an employer, extend the same courtesies, considerations, benefits, and protections to the important people in the lives of your single employees as you do to the spouses of your married employees. If you are a teacher, use examples and assign materials that highlight all the significant people in our lives, not just romantic partners. If you are a writer or an artist, feature friends in your creative work.

For People Who Are Intrigued by Single Life, But Have Concerns

If you have concerns about whether you would have friends who would be there for you if you committed to living single, you could try it out for a while. Adopt a single at heart mindset: invest in your friends, prioritize them, and be there for them. If you have been neglecting your friendships, it may take time to rebuild them or make new ones. Eventually, though, you will see if it pays off for you, not just with friends who show up for you, but also with greater self-esteem and a more fulfilling single life.

6

Our Kids, Other Kids, No Kids

I do not have kids, and never wanted any. I'm an only child, so I'm not an aunt or anything. I am completely happy with my childfree status.
—Laurie (thirty-five, Michigan)

The psychological pressures and cultural mandates that amass around parenting are strikingly similar to those that stalk our decisions about coupling. We—women especially—know we are supposed to want kids, just as we know we are supposed to yearn to be coupled. As single people, though, the kid question is a "damned if you do, damned if you don't" proposition. We are supposed to have kids (so it is bad if we don't), but we are supposed to do so with a spouse (so it is bad if we do). Fortunately, the single at heart are not bandied about by the conventional wisdom about how we are supposed to live, so we persist in living authentically, deciding for ourselves what role, if any, children will play in our lives.

Not wanting to put a romantic partner at the center of our lives is a defining characteristic of people who are single at heart. But not wanting kids isn't. We who are single at heart are even less likely to have kids than other single people, but we include in our numbers people who have kids and people who don't, people for whom kids have a place of prominence in their roles as aunts, uncles, teachers, coaches, or mentors, people who have no interest whatsoever in anyone's children, and just about every other permutation.

~~Why don't you want kids?~~

Fixed it!

Why do you want kids?

No Kids

For some who are single at heart, such as Laurie, the kid question is a nonissue. They were never interested. "Children are not a big part of my life, and I prefer it that way," Evan (forty, San Francisco, California) told me. Anna (fifty-three, Fayetteville, Tennessee) said that she is just "not a kid person." Donna (forty-nine, Seattle, Washington) said, "I'm glad I didn't succumb to that societal pressure." Peggy (sixty-seven, Atlanta, Georgia) thinks she might have succumbed if she had married, "even though I really didn't deeply want children." I doubt that Steve (thirty-nine, Bolton, England) would have; he describes himself as "fiercely childfree."

Some people who are single at heart are not quite so sure about whether they want to have kids. When they decide against it, their reluctance to give up the solitude and the freedom they so cherish looms large. David (sixty-five, Austin, Texas) said:

> My parents, and especially my mother who made a career of [caring for] us, were so in favor of their children and so happily dedicated to us, to the work, and costs we represented for them, and to our larger family-at-large, that it seemed almost unthinkable not to replicate that paradigm myself. But I just did not belong on that path. If I had followed it, regardless, I believe I would have endured a different set of emotional griefs about the loss of my independence and the freedoms I now enjoy.
>
> Finding peace and joy with our decision requires a fair balancing of the emotional books. It is a true danger that we can become mired in contemplation of the losses of not having children without then also honoring and lauding the positive gains one has "traded for."

Andrea (twenty-nine, New York City) sees herself as a kid person. She loves kids and wants to have them in her life, but not at the expense of her solitude or the psychological richness of her single adult life:

> I was a summer sleepaway camp counselor for two years and *loved* my scouts! I have a strong instinct to empathize with kids and find the idea of child-raising theoretically interesting. But I also know that it would drain me (I love sleep and quiet alone time and having intelligent conversations and doing grown-up things!), and it's not a decision I could reverse. I've struggled with the conflict in my conviction that I *could* be a great mother, yet I don't *want* to be. I hope to be a "cool aunt" to my cousins' and friends' kids!
>
> It's hard for me to see my friends, who aren't even "kid people" the way I am, automatically resign themselves to have kids.

• • •

To be a girl in my sixth-grade class was a very special thing. Every day for one hour, while the teachers ate lunch, one of us would get to watch the kindergarteners out on the playground. We were each assigned our day for doing this. My friend Lynn loved watching the kindergarteners. She couldn't wait for her day. I didn't mind it, but I shared none of Lynn's enthusiasm. When my day rolled around, I told Lynn she could take my place.

After lunch, my teacher stood in front of the class and announced in her most disappointed voice, "Bella didn't watch the kindergarteners today. She didn't want to."

I was more explicitly and publicly shamed for not being interested in kids than I ever have been for not being interested in marriage. Maybe my teacher thought that, as a child, I was malleable. But MaryL (sixty-two, Los Angeles, California) was still getting ridiculed when she was a fully-grown adult:

> The era I grew up in if you weren't married by thirty and hadn't dropped a baby or two, something was wrong with you. This kind of thinking was especially brutal in the African American community. As one guy I was (briefly) seeing sneered, "What kind of black woman are you that you don't want to have a baby?!"

Sometimes women who share that they do not want kids are just not believed. Keturah Kendrick has never wanted children. In *No Thanks: Black, Female, and Living in the Martyr-Free Zone*, she explained that other people are skeptical. They think she will change her mind. They think she will regret her decision. She doesn't and she won't. In the book she asks, "How can I regret not having something I never wanted?"[213]

Carla (thirty-three, Essex, England) who has "never felt a maternal stirring" in her life, has been second-guessed by medical professionals for years. Broaching the topic of sterilization, she was once told that no, that wasn't a good idea because she might meet a man someday and he might want children. The website of the National Health Service of the United Kingdom, where Carla lives, makes it clear that she cannot count on getting the procedure if she wants it. "Your GP can refuse to carry out the procedure or refuse to refer you for it if they do not believe it's in your best interests," the site reveals, adding, "You may be more likely to be accepted for the procedure if you're over thirty and have had children."[214] But Carla doesn't want children; for her, that's the point.

Pressures to marry and have kids can make it hard for people who don't want either to realize there's nothing wrong with that. As I showed in Chapter 2, on coming to understand yourself as single at heart, it can take years of trying to fix ourselves with therapy or self-help books or forcing ourselves to persist at dating or marrying or even remarrying, before we accept ourselves for who we really are.

It doesn't always end there. We still know that what we want isn't what we are supposed to want. The temptation is to perform the socially expected role. Pretend we really are interested in finding someone, but we're just so busy. Effuse about the wonder of children. That will placate our friends, relatives, and acquaintances for a while and spare us from some difficult conversations. But it will do nothing to help the other people who really don't want a spouse or children, either, and would be comforted or emboldened to know there are more like-minded souls out there than they ever realized.

Flipping the Script

"Young women today, one reason why they are less likely to plan to have or adopt kids than their forbears is that their engagement in friendship networks and professional networks is a kind of substitute for the need to create a family of one's own."[215]
—Stewart Friedman, University of Pennsylvania Professor of Management

For women (and men) who do not want kids, there is no "need" to create a family of their own. To say that their friendship networks and their professional networks, which they may highly value, are mere "substitutes" for creating the family they do not even want is to get these people all wrong. It is also condescending. Imagine if Friedman had instead said: "Young women today, one reason why some of them plan to have or adopt kids is that their need to create a family of one's own is a kind of substitute for the engagement in friendship networks and professional networks that they do not have and may never have."

The good news for people who do not want to have kids and don't want to be badgered about it is that the pressure to have kids may be subsiding a bit. In many places around the world, the birth rate is declining, as adults have fewer kids or none at all.[216] Relatively younger adults are especially likely to have no children, or to say that they don't want to have kids. For example, a 2021 US Census Bureau report focusing on older adults showed that among those who were seventy-five and older, 11 percent had no biological children. For the youngest of the old, ages fifty-five to sixty-four, the rate was nearly double: 20 percent had no biological children.[217] The same pattern emerged in another survey of adults of childbearing age who were asked whether they wanted to have kids. Of those who were in their forties, 46 percent said they didn't want to have kids. Of the younger adults, ages eighteen to thirty-nine, an even greater number, 60 percent, said the same thing.[218]

The angst around not having kids also seems to be subsiding. In 2002, when women in their early forties who did not already have kids were asked how they would feel if they never did have any, 55 percent said it would hardly bother them at all. By 2013, that number jumped up to 67 percent.[219]

Our Role Models

My mother's best friend, Mary, was a role model to me all my life! She became a chemist at a time when women didn't have careers. She turned down at least one marriage proposal (and probably more). She traveled so much, and always on her own terms. I adored her! And when she left me a small amount of money in her will I knew *exactly* what to with it . . . [and] took my mother on the trip she'd always wanted to do, to Ireland and Scotland to follow our family history. I wouldn't be who I am today without Mary's shining example.

—Clare (forty-nine)

When I first started studying single people decades ago, I wanted to know how single people were viewed by others. My colleagues and I did a whole series of studies, involving hundreds of participants. What we found was mostly disappointing—lots of evidence that people typically bought into the stereotypes that single people are self-centered and envious, and not as mature or as well-adjusted as married people.[220] Social scientists who have studied adults who do not have children (whether single or coupled) have found similarly harsh judgments of them, compared to adults who are parents.[221] The people who have no children because they don't want children (childfree, rather than childless), just like the single people who are single because they want to be single, are viewed especially unkindly.[222]

The results of those studies, as with all studies from the social sciences, are based on the average or typical responses across all of the participants in the studies. Hidden among those typical responders are people who have very different views. Instead of looking down on single people with no kids, they look up to them. When I asked the members of the Community of Single People Facebook group to tell me about their role models, they shared one story after another about the single people who inspired them. Some, such as Clare (quoted in the "Role Model" box), developed a special relationship with their role models. Others admired them from afar and continued to think about them and effuse about them decades later. I think there is something special about these stories. They suggest that from an early age, some children are noticing adults who are not living a conventional life; those adults stay with them in their imaginations, letting them know that they too can live their most joyful, authentic, meaningful, and psychologically fulfilling lives.

I know it's coming. After I've finished a talk about single people and open the floor for questions, someone will thrust their hand into the air and announce that they have located the tragic flaw in my argument: if too many people are persuaded that single life is a fulfilling life, that will spell the end of the species.

It won't. Single people have been having sex and having babies since eternity. Even when sex outside of marriage was the topic of gossipy whispers and when single parenting was far more stigmatized than it is now, it was done. The misplaced concern reflects the long-standing conflation of being single with not having kids and being married with being married with children.

In a way, it is understandable. Empirically, marital status and parental status are connected. Single people are less likely than married people to have kids, and people who are single at heart are even less likely than other single people to have kids. Increasingly, though, more single people are having kids and more married people are not, so the link is weakening.

Our Kids

I decided to become a single parent and it was the right decision. I have loved it and would not want to be a coupled parent if I had to do it all over again. Being a single parent allowed me to create a dyad with my daughter that is all about us and only us. My child has consistency and stability that children with two parents will never know. She will never be a pawn in a power match between adults. She has never had to worry about her parents divorcing. We are supported by a village and our lives are full of love. I am so glad that I raised her by myself.

—Maria (fifty-two, Beverly, Massachusetts)

Maria's story of single parenting is a triumph over the relentless stereotyping and stigmatizing of single parents and their children that is a blight on the US, where she lives, and many other nations around the world. Maria is not just defending her single-parent family as just as good as a married-parent family, she is proclaiming that in some ways it is better. It is better for her child, who has consistency and stability and the love of a whole village, it is better for Maria, who has sole say over child-rearing decisions, and it is better for the bond between them.

Maria's teenage daughter is flourishing. She's an honors student, a musician, and a kind and brave friend who stood up for a fellow student who was being mistreated. When she did not get a part in a musical theater production she had her heart set on, she still worked hard on the production. She earns money at summer jobs and is great fun at parties.

Maria is flourishing too. She's a financially secure engineer with a nice car and a home that she owns. She volunteers in her daughter's schools, and she and her daughter have vacationed at Yellowstone, in the Caribbean, and in Italy. The village Maria has built for the two of them includes neighbors, friends from school and work, parents from the parent-teacher organization, and adults and kids who share the same interests they do.

Not all single parents can relate to Maria's story. The struggling single parent is not just a myth. Dr. Amy Andrada, a research associate at the University of Edinburgh in Scotland, is a scholar of stigma and single motherhood who has been conducting in-depth interviews of single mothers.[223] She is finding that about one in five of them experience single parenting as difficult and isolating. They are the ones who yearn for a partner. They want the love and support, and the dedicated co-parenting, that they hope will come with marriage or long-term coupling. Nearly three times as many single mothers are ambivalent. They relish the freedom they have as single parents, but they would also like the intimacy and support of a partner. That leaves the other one in five single mothers, and they sound most like the people I call single at heart. Their experiences, Dr. Andrada told me, "gave them a newfound faith in single parenting and they couldn't imagine having to negotiate parenthood with a partner."

They love their kids, but now they're stuck with some bloke.[224]
—Hattie Crisell, quoting an acquaintance in "The rise of the alpha single"

A half-century or so ago, it would have been rare for someone like Maria, who is not married, to have a child. In some places, such as China, India, and much of Africa, it is still rare. But in many other nations around the world, it has become commonplace. In the US in 2014, 40 percent of babies were born to unmarried mothers, a huge jump from fewer than 10 percent in 1964. In Scandinavian countries in 2014, more than half of babies were born to women who were not married, and in some Latin American nations, those numbers reached 60 percent or higher.[225]

Even with the rise of single parenting, women who have been single their whole lives are less likely to be mothers than women who have married. In 2018 in the US, 85 percent of all women who were nearing the end of their childbearing years were mothers; for those who had never married, 59 percent were mothers.[226] Sometimes, when adults don't have children, it is because they don't want children. In fact, when adults in the US (men and women, married and unmarried) say they don't intend to have children and are then asked why, the number one reason is that they just don't want children.[227]

A substantial number though—43 percent—do not intend to have children even though they do want children. Most often, that's because of medical or financial reasons. But right up there in the top three reasons is one more—they do not intend to have the kids they would like to have because they don't have a partner.[228] Maria's story is a triumph over that obstacle too. She didn't let it deter her. Other people who are single at heart have done the same, or plan to. Yogesh, (twenty-six, Karnal, India), for example, hopes to adopt.

There's nothing wrong with wanting to marry before having children. Many people want to have a partner in their lives and a co-parent for their children, and they truly believe it is what is best for their kids. The problem comes when single people feel unduly pressured to either marry or not have kids at all; they really want kids, so out of desperation, they commit to partners who just don't have the skills or temperament to be good, or even acceptable, partners or parents. We already know, from a whole program of research, that people who are afraid of being single have lower standards for romantic partners.[229] When they are searching not just for a spouse but also for a co-parent, they are potentially putting their future children at risk.

People considering single parenting may feel dissuaded by the often-repeated claims that the children of single parents just don't do as well in life as the children of married parents. Those claims are often exaggerations or misrepresentations of what the research really shows.[230] They are perpetuating the belief in the Magical Mythical Romantic Partner.

A review of 122 studies of families in twenty-nine nations showed that differences favoring the children of married parents, when there were any, were typically small.[231] Even then, the differences don't necessarily occur *because* the children have one single parent instead of two married parents. Often what matters most is financial security, and there is no difference at all if the children come from families that are faring similarly economically.[232] Some nations systematically advantage nuclear families in their policies and practices, while others do more to equalize the resources available to single-parent and two-parent families; in the latter nations, the children of single parents are less likely to be disadvantaged and may even do better in some ways.[233] Racism, classism, and singlism can matter too; the children of single parents sometimes struggle not because they are being raised by just one parent, but because they are stereotyped, stigmatized, ostracized, and targeted with discrimination.

Sweeping claims about the fate of the children of single parents typically ignore the evidence for their strengths and advantages. For example, a six-year study of the children from nearly twenty-eight thousand households in the UK found that the children who had been in a single-parent household, even just temporarily, did as well or even better than the children who never lived in a single-parent family. They were more satisfied with their lives, they felt more positively about their families, and they were less likely to have problematic relationships with their peers.[234]

Instead of just assuming that the number of parents is what would matter most to children, UCLA professor Rena Repetti and her colleagues took a different approach. They asked what kinds of family environments could prove risky to children's mental or physical health. After reviewing every relevant study, they concluded that the truly risky families were the ones "characterized by conflict and aggression and by relationships that are cold, unsupportive, and neglectful."[235] That's what mattered most, not whether the children were raised by one parent or two. When single people who want to have children feel that they have no choice but to commit to a partner, regardless of any reservations they may have, they may well be setting themselves up for just such cold and distant family dynamics.

Maria's daughter is a teenager, and yet, Maria is proud to say, her life is drama free. "Do we have emotionally charged conversations? Yes. Does my daughter come to me in a dramatic state? Heck yeah. Is there screaming and yelling and slamming doors? No. As a parent, it is my job to teach her how to work through emotions."

University of Cambridge professor Susan Golombok and her colleagues conducted an intensive study of fifty-one single-mother families and fifty-two two-parent families with four-to-nine-year-old children, all of whom had been conceived by donor insemination. The research team conducted interviews, observed the families, and administered questionnaires to the mothers, the children, and their teachers. The two kinds of families were about the same in most ways— for example, there were no differences in the quality of the parenting or in the adjustment of the children. There was one way, though, that the families did differ—there was less conflict between mothers and their children in the single-mother families.[236]

Not Looking and Better Off for It

There's a lot of pressure to give children in single parent households a "father figure." There were men in their lives: my dad, my sister's husband, friends, teachers, and their now grown cousins. But I think it would've been so much more detrimental to all three of us had I spent time and energy on trying to get remarried. The girls and I are really grateful that I never tried to find them a stepdad.

—April (forty-nine, Burbank, California)

Parents who are single at heart are not trying to find a romantic partner to put at the center of their lives and thus have great advantages over single parents who are actively searching for a partner. They don't need to devote massive amounts of time to finding that partner or developing a relationship. All that angst about whether to introduce partners to their kids, and if so, when to do it and how? Managing the complicated psychology of their children's reactions? Parents who are single at heart are spared from all that, as are their children.

Dr. Andrada, the scholar of single motherhood, is a single mother who was raised by a single mother. Her mother was constantly trying to repartner and brought a string of partners into their home. "Oh gawd, what a mess—for everyone," she said. Dr. Andrada enjoys intimate relationships and dates now and then. But keeping her romantic life separate from her parental life has always been paramount. "I thoroughly enjoy my incredible bond and relationship with my child. I wholly appreciate the fact that it hasn't been compromised by trying to maintain a romantic relationship on behalf of my child. It means our relationship is based on only us two—thus explaining our very close bond." Dr. Andrada has given her son the consistency she never had as a child. Maintaining a positive relationship with him has always been her main focus.

Maria is at a place in her life where she has little need or desire for sex. "I am not repelled by it; it just does not factor in the top twenty things that matter in my life. Men are like parsley on the dinner plate of my life: it's nice when it's there, but it does not add to the nutritional value of the plate. It is not missed when it is not there."

Intimacy and love come in many flavors beyond the romantic variety, and all of the single at heart mothers and their children have lots of love in their lives. Maria, for example, has different kinds of intimacy with different people—similar to the "emotionships" I described in the last chapter. "I have friends with whom I share my fears about being a mother. I have friends with whom I share my work concerns. I have friends to whom I bare my soul as a woman. I have other friends with whom I share my concerns about the planet. I am very intimate with each of those people, and I know they are with me." Maria and her daughter have each other's love, the love of their dogs, and the love of the many people in the village that Maria built for them. The two of them are huggers and voice their love often. "So our lives are full of love, support, and (equally important) people who lovingly point out where we can do better," she shared.

Can You Be a Single Parent and Have Your Freedom Too?

I'm happier than I've ever been. Even when I was broke and ghostwriting op-eds to buy groceries, I was happy because I was finally free.[237]
—Lyz Lenz, "The Subversive Joy of Being a Single Mother"

Freedom is at the heart of what the single at heart love about their single lives. I thought they might see parenting as a constraint on their freedom, one that they abided because it was outweighed by what they loved about raising their children on their own. But when I asked, "As a single parent, do you feel that you have freedom in your life?" they instead said that they reveled in their freedom. As single parents, they get to be the deciders—something the single at heart value—and they use their freedom to create psychologically rich lives for themselves and their children.

Maria said, "As a single parent, I have an incredible amount of freedom. I see my coupled friends who have to negotiate a trip, for example. I, on the other hand, just find a sitter and I am gone. Moreover, I am able to do what I want with my daughter. For April vacation, we are renting an RV and driving through thirteen states. Just my daughter, my dogs, and me."

Dr. Andrada said, "I've realized how blessed I am to not have to negotiate my child's welfare (or mine) with another person. Because of this I have been able to study abroad, take jobs in other countries, work internationally, and travel/explore—all with my son by my side."

The single parents who were once married are especially enthusiastic about their newfound freedom. Lyz Lenz, who said she is happier than she had ever been, had left a marriage. April (forty-nine, Burbank, California), a single mother who also had been married previously, said of her life as a single parent, "It's the most free I've ever felt."

The single at heart are free spirits, living their most authentic lives, even when that makes them different. That too can be compatible with single parenting. Maria put it this way: "I have never been afraid to be different. Becoming an engineer as a woman is not for those who like the well-worn path. Being different means I am willing to take a risk and figure it out as I go along. At the end of the day, that is the essence of parenting."

Can You Be a Single Parent and Have Solitude Too?

When my daughter goes off to a sleepover, I don't go out with anyone. I love to just enjoy the house all to myself.
—Maria (fifty-two, Beverly, Massachusetts)

Securing precious alone time was a challenge for single at heart parents when their children were very young. Some got almost no solitude at all. But they figured out ways to carve out some time to themselves, and as their kids got older, that got easier. Dr. Andrada said, "For a long time there was *no time* to myself, because I was constantly working and running about (one-woman team). But as my son has gotten older, and I've become more financially stable and built my communities, I find *lots* of time to do things, such as the gym, activities, hanging with friends, and even reading a damn book (that's not for work)." Maria said that "raising a kid means giving up a lot of personal time." But once her daughter was old enough for sleepovers, she had that time to herself. She also gets a massage at least once a month.

I first interviewed April years ago when her two daughters were in their early teens. They understood how important it was to their mom to have some time to herself, but they weren't just humoring her—they also appreciated having some privacy. In their two-bedroom apartment, after dinner, each of the girls might retreat to a bedroom, and April would stay in the living room. That way, they each got a measure of solitude and privacy. Other times they would all gather in the living room and find solitude together: "We'll each have on our own headphones: Sylvia learning a dance routine on YouTube, Riley watching a TV show or movie, and me listening to a podcast." Interspersed with their quiet times were more raucous happenings; "Sometimes we'll throw a dance party in the living room or break out in song together."

About Those Supposedly Frazzled Single Mothers

Frankly, I don't know how women do it with husbands.
—April (forty-nine, Burbank, California)

When Iris (sixty-five, Portugal) was nineteen, she was told that she was sterile. Kids were not part of her life plan. She was married briefly—twice—when she was young, and learned that she was pregnant while finishing her PhD. She gave birth and landed a university job at thirty-six, newly single again. This time she remained single and never lived with a partner again.

"I think subsistence farming is probably easier than raising a kid alone as an assistant professor," she said. Nonetheless, she filled her daughter's life with joy. "When she was little, I took her everywhere—camping, Mt. Laguna, Catalina Island, Golden Gate Park, Rockies, Chicago, all over Europe. The two of us were a family. Christmas was fun because I knew what she wanted, and she was happy and safe." Now, Iris said, "I cannot imagine the universe without my daughter."

What would Iris have imagined if she realized she could get pregnant? Without a husband to help, would she expect to feel more harried, sleep-deprived, and burdened by the household chores that she alone would have to handle? Would she anticipate sacrificing time with her child and any fun for herself as she did all the work of providing for her family?

That's the standard story about single motherhood, and not just in the popular press. In their help center, the American Psychological Association provides a dedicated section on single parenting. "The single parent may feel overwhelmed by the responsibilities of juggling caring for the children, maintaining a job, and keeping up with the bills and household chores," the organization cautioned.[238]

But just how disadvantaged are single mothers, relative to married mothers? The sociologist Joanna R. Pepin and two colleagues analyzed data from ten years of American Time Use Surveys. Their nationally representative sample included more than twenty-three thousand single (not married) and married mothers. The married mothers were all married to a man.[239]

The researchers found that some of the mothers were in fact "time poor"—the married ones. Married mothers spent more time cleaning, cooking, shopping, and doing laundry than the single mothers. They also got less sleep and had less fun. All that, and they spent no more time caring for their children than the single mothers. The social scientists tested several explanations for their findings and settled on one that seemed to fit best: the married mothers were performing the role of the good wife and good mother.

It's not that mothers don't benefit from having another adult around. They do, as long as it is not a husband. For example, the mothers who lived with extended family members such as grandparents or aunts spent less time on both housework and childcare.

The results came as a surprise to many readers who learned about the study from an op-ed in the *Washington Post*, but not to Lara Bazelon. In an article for Slate, she wrote:

> Count me in as a single mom who is not at all surprised.
> Divorce, as it turns out, can bring freedom not only from
> a broken relationship but from the day-to-day grind that is

the performance of motherdom. There is no need to be seen as constantly cooking, bathing, doing laundry, and cleaning up when no one is watching.

There's also less need to spend a bunch of time nagging—not the kids, but their dad.[240]

At the end of her essay, Bazelon shared, "When people ask me if I plan to get married again or even live with someone else, my response is very direct—hell, no."[241][i]

Maria did not know anything about that study when she told me that she is often asked how she has time for all the volunteer work she does in her daughter's school. She always replies that she and her daughter have time for the things that matter to them. "In fairness," she added, "I am lucky enough to be able to afford a housekeeper who cleans my house, so that does help. But I honestly think that not having a husband frees up my time far more so."

Of the different categories of single mothers in the study—divorced, cohabiting, and never married—the greatest advantage went to those who had always been single. They were especially likely to do less housework than the married mothers, and to spend more time sleeping and enjoying some leisure.

The Successful Single Parent

Mothers who enjoyed single motherhood the most and relished its opportunities and benefits often had a very strong sense of self and independence. They maintained communities and sought out new groups/ people to share experiences with—as single people and as parents. They were open to exploring new areas and activities. And made considerable headway toward reevaluating family and gender norms—often focusing on what best suited them and their kids, rather than what was socially expected of them.

—Dr. Amy Andrada

Dr. Andrada is describing single mothers who sound a lot like people who are single at heart. That "strong sense of self and independence" is the quintessential single at heart spirit. In designing a life that worked best for them and their children, rather than following the expected life script, they were living authentically, something that the single at heart value tremendously. And in exploring new things, they were creating the kinds of psychologically rich lives that the single at heart prize.

I'm not any kind of parent and never wanted to be. If I were a single parent, though, I think I would be tempted to focus solely on my kids and on the work I'd need to do to support them. For me, just managing those two huge things would already be daunting. Although I would not be proud of myself for it, I'd probably let other things slide, such as the time I spend with friends or my communities. I'd give up on having an identity outside of my family.

But according to Dr. Andrada, that would not be a path to flourishing. Of course single parents need economic resources, such as money to pay the bills and afford activities for the kids, so they need to devote time to their work life, but it is also important to build social and community resources. Solo parenting can feel isolating, and the stigma attached to it compounds that potential difficulty. Maintaining ties with friends and other supportive people and communities can be a great antidote. Communities of other single people or single parents can sometimes provide the kind of support that no one else can. One other thing is significant too, Dr. Andrada said: "Have an identity outside of your children and family—and keep it. Cultivate it. And work to maintain it."

The single at heart parents who were flourishing were doing just what Dr. Andrada recommended. For example, April and her daughters love the theater, and the supportive people in their lives include their theater friends as well as other friends from work and school, April's parents, and her sister. April's community involvement started with joining the parent-teacher association and then saying yes to every opportunity that arose.

She wrote grants. She joined the boards of nonprofit organizations. Most importantly, looking to bond with other single parents, she began blogging about her experiences as a single parent. She joined an LA moms' blog. As she reports, "Within a year, blogging had become a huge part of my life." April has become friends with fellow bloggers and their families have socialized together. April also has her work identity—she's a paralegal. When I asked her to describe herself, her answer began with this: "Single mom, theater lover, paralegal, blogger, board member." April had developed social and community resources, and she had an identity outside of her family.

I asked Dr. Andrada, who is Latinx, if she wanted to address other Latinx single parents. She said, "We as Latinx people should cultivate a sense of self and identity by and for ourselves. And wholly cultivate community engagements—both in and outside Latinx spaces. As Hispanic/Latinx people we have to negotiate the roles of women as parents and as people, especially in how we are taught to be always in service to others—often at the cost of ourselves." Dr. Andrada also noted that Latinx single-parent families are among the families that are at special risk of being stigmatized: "It is vital that we reexamine how race plays a part in our notions as single people and single parents—especially within the US."

Our Role Models

I saw two adults treating each other with love, respect, and humor. I saw that it was possible to be a whole, healthy adult without marriage and, in my aunt's case, without biological children of one's own.[242]
—Dani McClain, describing her single mother and aunt who raised her, in
We Live for the We: The Political Power of Black Motherhood

The term "single parent" can obscure another key to successful single parenting. Single parents are not always raising their children single-handedly. April, for example, has had lots of help from her parents. In *We Live for the We: The Political Power of Black Motherhood*, Dani McClain explained that she was raised by her mother, who had never married, in a household that also included her maternal aunt. Both women lavished Dani with love and attention. Dani and her mother also had the support of "othermothers" such as Dani's grandmother, great-grandmother, other aunts, and elders from the community.[243]

During their teenage years, which can be trying for both the teens and their parents, children raised by single mothers in extended-family households do especially well. In a comprehensive study, more than eleven thousand US teens were followed for six years. They came from ten different kinds of households, including those headed by married parents, cohabiting parents, single mothers, single fathers, and divorced and never-married single mothers in multigenerational households. The children of the divorced mothers in mutigenerational households did just as well as the children of married parents. The teens raised in multigenerational households by mothers who had always been single did even better than the teens raised by married parents. They were less likely to drink or smoke, and more of them graduated from high school and enrolled in college.[244]

Singlism and the Single-Parent Family

When I sent my daughter to summer camp, I had to send a certified copy of her birth certificate when others didn't.
—Maria (fifty-two, Beverly, Massachusetts)

In places such as the US, where skeptical attitudes toward single-parent families still prevail, single parents and their children are at risk for being stereotyped, stigmatized, marginalized, and targeted with discrimination. That's true of all single-parent families, not just the single at heart. Sometimes disadvantages are written right into the laws of the land. Maria pointed out, "As a single mother, I pay a higher tax rate than if I had a stay-at-home spouse providing free childcare and housekeeping." She feels fortunate that she can afford it. Her economic security stands in defiance of the stereotype of single mothers as uniformly destitute. When she wanted to buy a large home, one realtor after another showed her only small ones, insisting that was all she needed. She now owns the home she wanted and has been asked repeatedly whether it is something she got in her divorce. (She has never been married.) She has also dealt with insinuations that she can only afford her lifestyle because of child support.

Maria's daughter hated class assignments to make a Father's Day card. When she told her teachers she didn't have a father, sometimes they would tell her to make it for her grandfather or uncle. But she didn't have any grandfathers or uncles either. Eventually, she came up with a solution: she just wrote "Dad" on the card, then told her mom she did that because of the teacher, but the card was actually for her. In the end, Maria said, "she learned the life skill of picking her battles and finding her power in the situation."

When Dr. Andrada's son was little, long before Amy had become a scholar of stigma and single parenthood, he asked her a heartbreaking question, "Mama, why don't the little boys play with me?" They did play with him, on his soccer and baseball teams and during karate lessons, but he wasn't invited to the birthday parties or sleepovers. Amy was excluded too—she wasn't part of the friendship networks of the other moms, but she didn't think much of it at the time. She was just worried about her son. She tried everything she could think of. She encouraged her son to be more outgoing and friendly. She enlisted other family members to show up at her son's games. She changed her own style, dressing first more conservatively, then more provocatively. Nothing helped. Utterly frustrated, she vented to a coworker, who asked her whether all the other mothers were married. They were. Fake it, he suggested. Put a ring on your finger. Amy was incredulous, but nothing else had worked, so she bought a cheap imitation of a diamond ring and put it on her ring finger. "Then . . . BAM! *Everything changed.* My son started to be invited to activities with his teammates and peers. Other mothers who had seen me for months, even years, began approaching me as if we had been longtime friends."

All the single parents I've talked to, for this single at heart project and previous projects, wish their children had been spared from the stigmatizing treatment they sometimes received. When Amy's son was getting excluded from the after-school parties and gatherings with the other boys his age, she said that "the thought that, in some way, I was responsible for my son being denied anything hurt me in the deepest way." That hurt motivated Amy to pursue her graduate education and become a social scientist. She is exposing the psychological dynamics and the historical and cultural contexts of the stigmatizing of single parents and their children, in her quest for greater fairness for her son and all of the children of single parents.

It can be especially hard for the children of single parents, and their parents, when the children are young. Over time, though, when they have parents like Maria, Amy, and April, they develop a more sophisticated understanding of the world and an appreciation for their life experiences. Amy's son has seen her study, work internationally, and travel too. He "has witnessed for himself that families come in all shapes and sizes." He knows that what matters most is not the number of parents a child has, but "a parent's commitment to their child, and whether we have support in our community." April said that her kids are "totally aware of the stupid things people say" about single-parent families, "but they consider our family a success story."

Maria has become a heroine not just to her daughter, but to her daughter's high school friends, who call Maria a badass. One of those friends wants to be just like Maria—an engineer who is not married.

The Joy of Single Parenting

I feel proud and empowered and grateful and lucky and pure joy!
—April (forty-nine, Burbank, California)

The utter joy of single parenthood is the story none of the single parents in my research had ever heard. They all had to discover it for themselves, often to their great surprise. When April shared that she felt "proud and empowered and grateful and lucky and pure joy," it was in a blog post declaring, "I'm a homeowner!"[245] April's first rental after leaving her marriage was a one-bedroom apartment, furnished with hand-me-downs, where she slept on a futon in the living room so her girls could have the bedroom. At the time she had not graduated from college. Now she has a college degree, a paralegal's certificate, and has worked her way up to the managerial level at an esteemed company. She has some other achievements too: "Trustee of my own estate plan. And holder of my own deed. And future."

Dr. Andrada was also surprised by how her life turned out. "I started out poor, a product of a single-parent family, the daughter of an immigrant, and a mixed bag of race, ethnicity, and religion." She has been especially heartened by the bond she developed with her son. Referencing times before she began her studies, she told me, "I could have never imagined such a fulfilling and positive relationship. And though extremely difficult in the beginning (poverty, isolation, stigma, etc.), we have weathered it all and still have a healthy, productive, and unbreakable bond."

Maria was already a mature adult who "had put a heck of a lot of work" into herself when she had her daughter at thirty-five. She was financially secure too. She's been joyfully single throughout the entire experience—before her daughter was born, while raising her, and now, as her daughter is on the cusp of adulthood. "I enjoyed being single and pregnant," she told me. And raising her daughter by herself has been a "thoroughly enjoyable experience."

"I will never remarry," Lyz Lenz proclaimed at the end of her essay on the subversive joy of being a single mother. "I love my freedom too much."[246]

Other Kids

I never wanted to marry and never did marry. I have five hundred children. They all graduated from the bookstore.[247]

—Emoke B'Racz, former owner of a bookstore in Asheville, North Carolina

Many people like Emoke B'Racz, who never wanted to marry, never did marry, and never had kids of their own, are meaningfully connected to other children. B'Racz nurtured bonds with the hundreds of children (and adults) who frequented the bookstore she opened when she came to the US from Hungary. She told her local public radio station that the bookstore was never a business; instead, "It's more living a good life and healing people who come to the store by giving them good stuff."[248]

Other people who have no kids of their own are devoted to other children in roles such as teachers, coaches, librarians, therapists, social workers, medical professionals, religious and spiritual leaders, nannies, and camp counselors. Examples from people who are single at heart include Carmela (forty-four, Nayarit, Mexico), who is a teacher; Sonya (forty-seven, Parkersburg, West Virginia), who is a teacher and a librarian; and Andrea (twenty-nine, New York City), who was a camp counselor. Even Steve (thirty-nine, Bolton, England), who calls himself "fiercely childfree," volunteers at a parkrun; "I fully understand that children need some degree of structured play to develop and thrive," he explained.

For some people with no children, their connections to other children are personal rather than professional. They are the older siblings, the doting aunts and uncles, the honorary aunts and uncles to the children of their friends, and the godparents. Liz (sixty, Washington, DC) said, "I am very attached to my nieces and nephew and my grandniece. I have always been a favorite aunt, who the nieces confided in. I get along well with my friends' children." MaryL (sixty-two, Los Angeles, California) is also "the favorite aunt in the family." Amy (forty-four, Frisco, Texas) is delighted to be able to make it to all of her nieces' and nephews' sports games. These adults can model a different way of being in the world and a different way of thinking than what those children see in their own parents or other parents. They can be confidants, mentors, special friends, and sources of emotional and sometimes financial support.

In *Childfree by Choice*, Dr. Amy Blackstone points out that people without children are not reproducing biologically, but they are engaging in "social reproduction." They are carrying out "roles, actions, and responsibilities required for helping our fellow humans become participating and contributing members of society."[249]

If this were a conventional book about single people, I'd make a big deal out of this section. I'd say something like, "See, single people who don't have kids still love kids and dedicate themselves to them! We are the ones showing up at their games, the fun aunts and uncles, and the people they turn to when no one else seems to understand them. We're helping their parents too." In many instances, such as the ones I've already described, all that would be true. The problem comes when people with no kids feel obligated to make a show of their love of children, even when they are actually not all that interested. Being single at heart is about living authentically. That means owning all of our life choices. There's nothing special about faking it.

Advice For the Single at Heart

If you don't have kids because you don't want kids, feel proud of yourself for resisting the pressure to follow a path that doesn't suit you. Own your authentic childfree life.

If you do have kids, proudly own that too. If it suits your personality, boast about your children as effusively as any other parent. Treat yourself just as kindly as partnered parents treat themselves—hire that babysitter if you can and do something you enjoy. Dr. Andrada, a single parent and a scholar who has studied single parents, offers these two suggestions: "It is an honor to raise your kid—with it just being you two. Act like it," and "It's a freedom unlike most things you will experience. Appreciate it."

If the important kids in your life include people such as your students, children you mentor or coach, or your nieces and nephews, don't let anyone ever tell you that you are not making substantial contributions to the next generation.

For Our Allies

If your single friends have kids in their lives, including in their roles such as teachers and coaches, show the same interest in them as you would in anyone else's kids. If they don't have kids and you do, don't let that be grounds for excluding them from social events; welcome the opportunity, with them around, to have wide-ranging conversations that are not so focused on kids.

If you are coupled and have children and your single friends or acquaintances have kids too, be sure their children are included in playdates and parties just as often and as warmly as any other children. Be sure the single parents are not excluded from the grown-up gatherings either.

Dr. Andrada has this to say about single-mother families: "Do not treat them as if their family type is a consequence of poor decisions. It is often the exact opposite—it has been very well thought-out, intentional, and often the best choice for her and her children." Also remember that some single-parent families are the result of the death of a parent.

It is wise and kind to keep in mind that people have very different experiences and wishes with regard to the role of children in their lives. Beware of assuming that all adults (and especially women) want and will eventually have kids. Remember that some people who do not have kids may have wanted them very badly (and they have already considered the options you may be tempted to suggest, such as adoption). Others may not be interested in children at all—they don't want children of their own and they may or may not find it enjoyable to be around children. If you are an educator, encourage your students to imagine and value all different kinds of life paths. If you are a medical professional or a mental health professional, listen carefully to your patients and clients, so you can hear what they really want and not just what you think they should want. If you are an employer or a policymaker, keep in mind that many people provide care to adults, not just to children, and they should be supported too.

For People Who Are Intrigued by Single Parenting, But Have Concerns

If you want to have kids but worry that it will be too difficult to have children as well as the kind of single life that you crave, remember that many who are single at heart are already doing so successfully. Keep in mind that alongside all the challenges you may face, you will also have some rarely recognized advantages, such as the ones I discussed in this chapter.

Dr. Andrada suggests this: "Ask yourself one question: what do *you* want? Not what is expected from you."

Dani McClain's perspective, described in *We Live for the We: The Political Power of Black Motherhood*, is also a wise one: "Throughout my thirties, I was sympathetic, but somewhat baffled, as I watched some of my women friends struggle to make peace with their unmarried, unpartnered status. Many of them seemed to feel that kids were unlikely, since no partner was in sight, but their predicaments just looked to me like another way to do life."[250] Do your life in the way you find most authentic and fulfilling.

7

Intimacy

What subculture is going to take up the mantle of being the proud
queer place that resists the idea that all intimacies are about true love,
romance, marriage, lifelong commitment, and monogamy?
—Pamela Haag, Big Think, "The UnQueered World:
Take a Walk on the Mild Side"[251]

I have an answer to Pamela Haag's question: the single at heart are going to
take up that mantle. Thinking about intimacy, and practicing intimacy, in
bigger, broader ways that transcend the conventions of romance and marriage
are at the heart of who we are. To us, having a life that is not organized
around a conventional monogamous relationship with a romantic partner is
freeing. We get to follow our hearts, enjoying intimacy on our own terms, in
ways that bring us joy and enrich our lives.

We live in happy defiance of the pressures of compulsory coupling, that
way of thinking that regards coupled life as a more natural and normal life,
superior to single life. We have little tolerance for compulsory heterosexuality
either. The single at heart are less likely to be heterosexual than people who are
not single at heart. In the single at heart quiz, 90 percent who scored as clearly
not single at heart identified as heterosexual, compared to 72 percent of those
who clearly were single at heart. But even those among us who are heterosexual
roll our eyes at the notion that heterosexuality is normal and natural and
superior to everything else. We don't buy into compulsory sexuality either.
People who are single at heart are more likely than those who are not single
at heart to be asexual ("ace"), a person who experiences little or no sexual
attraction. In the quiz, 3 percent who were not single at heart identified as
asexual, compared to 12 percent of those who were single at heart. Again,

though, even the 88 percent of us who are not asexual are unlikely to think that experiencing sexual attraction is more natural or normal than not experiencing it, or that people who are sexual are superior to those who are asexual.

I know that the story I am telling about intimacy is not what the conventional wisdom would have us believe. I realize that the skeptics reading this chapter will expect to find that intimacy is the downfall of the single at heart. They probably assume that without a romantic partner anchoring our lives, we are sexually frustrated, that we feel deprived of romance, and starved for love.

I gave the single at heart people who shared their life stories with me every opportunity to say that intimacy was a problem for them. I asked open-ended questions, such as "Is there anything you don't like about living single? Anything from the world of committed romantic coupling that you wish you had?" I asked if they had intimacy in their lives. I asked if they had love in their lives. I also asked about their sexual history, and I specifically asked if they considered themselves asexual or aromantic (a person who experiences little or no romantic attraction). In the single at heart quiz, I asked, "Think about the possibility that when you go to sleep at night, there might not be anyone else in bed with you. How does that make you feel?"

The takeaway was clear. It was rare for sex or romance to be described as an issue by people who are single at heart. Some weren't interested. Others were quite interested and found ways to fulfill their needs without following the standard script that puts a monogamous romantic partner solely in charge of satisfying intimacy. We who are single at heart think about intimacy in expansive ways that go beyond the bonds of the conventional. Don't try to tell us that romantic love is the only love that counts.

In most studies of sex and sexual satisfaction, single people are never asked whether they want to be single. When they are asked, their answer turns out to matter quite a lot. A study of nearly twenty-five hundred German adults uncovered evidence of sexual disappointment among single people—but it was mostly among the singles who wished they had a romantic partner. The single people who were not looking for a partner were about as sexually satisfied as the married people.[252]

Sex in the life of the single at heart offers a world of possibilities. Without a romantic partner who expects to be prioritized, we have more freedom to have

different kinds of sex (not limited by what a conventional partner might want),
different amounts of sex (including none), and to have it when and if we want
it. In theory, people with a committed romantic partner have easier access to
sex, particularly if they live with that person. And sometimes that's true. But
other times, that access is no more real than the Magical Mythical Romantic
Partner. Being coupled does not mean that you and your partner always want
the same kind of sex or the same amount of sex, or that the timing of your
interest in sex is always perfectly aligned, or that the sex is any good. Even
when having a romantic partner does bring easier access to good sex, it can
also come with complications, as, for example, when you become sexually
attracted to someone else without feeling free to pursue that possibility.

Easy access can mean not just that sex and romantic partnership are
available, but also that they are expected to take center stage. That is just
what the single at heart don't want: a sexual or romantic partnership to steal
away the time or love we want to devote to the other people or pursuits that
bring meaning, richness, and joy to our lives.

We are comfortable with the intimacy in our lives because we are
following our hearts. We define intimacy on our own more expansive terms.
Our intimacy is authentically our own. That's why the place of intimacy in
our lives is not our downfall, but one of our strengths.

Our Sex Lives

I love being head over heels for someone, and it's such a fun time to
explore sexual chemistry and all that. I adore having emotionally close,
loving relationships. I also love my social community and my own space.
I like having the freedom to take off without having to check in with
people or have someone keep tabs on me. I'm just very independent and
have always been happier without conventionally entangled/enmeshed
relationships. In typical monogamous language, I prefer "casual"
relationships and have no desire to cohabitate, join finances, get married, etc.

—Alyssa (twenty-seven, Los Angeles, California)

Alyssa, who identifies as a lesbian, has happily incorporated fun sex and emotionally close relationships into her life without putting a monogamous relationship partner at the center of it. She has sex, love, and her freedom too. She is happy not to have those continual check-ins with a partner that so many people who are not single at heart find so comforting.

When Alyssa said that she has no interest in cohabiting, joining finances, or getting married, she was telling us that she is not interested in riding what author Amy Gahran has called "the relationship escalator."[253] That's the typical expectation about how a romantic relationship will progress, from the initial contact and courtship, though identifying as a couple and establishing routines of togetherness, then onto the commitment to a long-term future, the merging of home and finances, and finally getting legally married and maybe having kids too. When Alyssa begins dating someone, she lets them know early on that she is not interested in monogamy or enmeshment.

A number of people who shared their single at heart life stories described similar preferences. Evan (forty, San Francisco, California), who is gay, said, "I sometimes go on dates, although I never do so with the expectation or intention that a committed long-term relationship will develop. I think it can be fun to meet new people, hear about other people's lives, etc." Donna (forty-nine, Seattle, Washington), who is heterosexual, said, "I have had a *lot* of relationships and short-term encounters that would have been hard to do in the frame of monogamy." Iris (sixty-five, Portugal) said, "Everyone hates bisexuals, but I truly am interested in the more androgynous of both sexes." Twice in her life, she experienced what she called "out of control love," adding, "I will happily think of them on my deathbed, but you couldn't pay me to live with either one."

There is a name for the openness to a number of meaningful relationships without prioritizing one person as the primary partner: solo polyamory. In Haili Blassingame's essay for the *New York Times*'s "Modern Love," Blassingame shared, "I liked how solo polyamory cherished and prioritized autonomy and the preservation of self, and I found its rejection of traditional models of romantic love freeing." Her choice, she added, was "to be single and not looking but very much loving."[254]

Jesica, a thirty-eight-year-old from Los Angeles, California, who is straight, had one long-term romantic relationship more than a decade ago, but it was not very satisfying. She is "sexually open-minded and loves to explore:"

> I have also gotten into the BDSM [bondage, discipline (or domination), sadism (or submission), and masochism] life-style and have had a lot of different experiences with different kinds of men. I went through a period of just casual sexual encounters and now I am at a stage in my life where I prefer more connection and substance than just sex with a man. At this point, I prefer men that are familiar with the lifestyle as well, not just "vanilla" relationships anymore.

As a single person, Jesica got to honor her sexual open-mindedness and her love of exploration. She tried out different experiences as her tastes and preferences evolved, without fear of judgment from a conventional romantic partner.

For some people who are single at heart and enjoy sex, a "friends with benefits" relationship might work well. The single at heart aren't going to complain about a sexual relationship that "isn't going anywhere;" that may be just what they want. At the same time, they typically value their friends, and might enjoy having sex in a relationship with all the fun and companionship and caring that friendship has to offer.

In informal conversations and online discussions over the years, single people who are interested in sex but not a serious romantic relationship (not all of whom are single at heart) have also mentioned casual sexual partners, booty calls, and escorts. Some look for people in open marriages or in other consensually nonmonogamous relationships. Some use dating apps, clearly specifying what they do and do not want.

Our Role Models

My aunt, Harriet "Hat" McAdams, was born in 1930, the eldest of seven children in an Irish Catholic family. At that time and in that culture, the only "acceptable" options for women were marriage and motherhood or becoming a nun. Neither suited Hat. She never married, she worked full-time in office roles, and she lived an adventurous life. She learned to pilot an airplane, crew a yacht, and she traveled internationally. Hat was elegant, kind, generous, and loving. She had many friends, and she often helped friends and family. To commemorate Hat, each year I make a point of doing something adventurous, brave, or generous that Hat would have done. These are my "Hat tricks." So far they've included a few international trips, writing and publishing a book, managing to purchase a home (no small feat as a self-employed writer), and making big efforts to help people in need. Like me, Hat was not conventionally "single." She did engage in long-term, deep romantic relationships, but she chose not to live with, marry, or merge finances with her partners. In my own life, I evolved to adopt the "solo" style of polyamory—which means I'm open to having more than one deeply intimate relationship at a time, just without exclusivity and without merging my identity or life infrastructure with any intimate partner. Hat's relationships were probably monogamous, but the way she retained her autonomy and authenticity was a strong influence in my own approach to life and love.
—Amy Gahran, author of *Stepping Off the Relationship Escalator: Uncommon Love and Life*

People who are single at heart don't put a romantic partner at the center of their lives in part because there is so much more they want to do with their lives than prioritize a partner. Some do want sex and the intimacy that can come with it. But they also want that part of their lives to stay in its place, so they still have all the time they want to devote to the other people in their lives and their other important pursuits. Andrea (twenty-nine, New

York City) found a solution that worked well for her when she was in college—hookup culture. Here's how she described her hookups:

> We only interacted between 2 a.m. and 6 a.m., and there was vulnerable conversation (which I valued) in addition to sex. I was aware that I was supposed to feel unsatisfied with this arrangement, but I was actually 100 percent content with it. The compartmentalization left me with uncompromised free time to study, participate in clubs, and hang out with friends.

Laurie (thirty-five, Michigan) loves the freedom single life gives her to pursue her passions without ever having to justify that to anyone. She runs half and full marathons, with a goal of doing at least a half marathon in every state. Her biggest passion, though, is horses. She's been riding since she was a child and has won a national championship. When she was younger, she had a serious romantic relationship. It was what she thought she was supposed to do:

> I like the companionship that comes with a relationship—to a point. Although I liked, perhaps loved, my boyfriend, I didn't want to get married or commit more time to the relationship. I always felt like I had to fiercely protect my "me" time, but also tended to feel guilty about how I spent my time. If I'm spending time with my boyfriend, I'm not spending it with family or horses. If I'm not spending it with the boyfriend, I'm a bad girlfriend.

Laurie was relieved when that relationship ended. She thought a lot about her life and read about the possibilities that single life could offer. She had experienced the kind of intimate relationship that a lifetime of conditioning had told her she *should* want. Instead she found that it stood in the way of what she really did love. Eventually, she said, "It clicked: I don't have to keep pursuing what I don't want. It's OK to be happy as a single person. The burden was lifted." Her story illustrates just one reason why some people who are single at heart don't have much sex or romance in their lives. There are others too.

Our Not-So-Sexual Lives

Angela Chen, author of *Ace: What Asexuality Reveals About Desire, Society, and the Meaning of Sex*, wrote that she did not know what it felt like: "To think about sex at all when I was alone. To feel any physical urge for sex distinct from wanting the emotional intimacy it created."[255]

As she came to understand what it meant to be asexual, she realized, "what I had passed off as sexual attraction even to myself was something else entirely: aesthetic appreciation, a desire for emotional and physical closeness, a certain possessiveness."[256]

Some people just don't experience sexual attraction. It's not because they are depressed, taking some medication that messes with their libido, or because they just haven't yet met anyone hot enough. They are asexuals, or "aces"—the A in LGBTQIA+ (lesbian, gay, bisexual, transgender, queer, intersex, and asexual). On Twitter, @AsexualsNet quipped, "To people who 'don't get' asexuality: Think of someone you aren't attracted to. Now imagine that is how you feel about everyone. The end."[257]

Asexuality exists on a spectrum, so it can be a bit more complicated than never feeling sexually attracted to anyone. A demisexual, for example, according to a succinct definition by Michael Gold in the *New York Times*, "generally does not experience sexual attraction unless they have formed a strong emotional, but not necessarily romantic, connection with someone."[258] It is not as simple as not ever having sex either. Some asexuals have sex for reasons unrelated to sexual attraction—for example, to please a partner. It is possible to experience little or no sexual attraction to any other person and still have a sex drive. Some asexuals experience sexual arousal that is not tied to sexual attraction to a particular person and enjoy masturbating.

Some admire particular bodies—the aesthetics of them, not their sex appeal. Many want and enjoy emotionally intimate relationships. Like other kinds of people who are single at heart, asexuals realize that intimacy is about much more than just sex.[259]

The study of the sexual satisfaction of nearly twenty-five thousand Germans showed that, on average, the single people who were not pining for a partner wanted to have sex less frequently than the single people who wished they were coupled.[260] Maybe that's because people who like being single include a disproportionate number who are asexual.

When I wrote my first book, *Singled Out*, I had never heard of asexuality. Now it is a social movement with websites, conferences, forums, celebrations, attention from the media and from scholars, and, most importantly, pride. Today's out-and-proud asexuals aren't about to be shamed by anyone. They know that asexuality is normal and natural, and that it can be divine.

In a finding that came as a shock to many, Americans have been having *less* sex over time. That was the conclusion of an analysis of the sexual behavior of more than twenty-six thousand adults from 1989 through 2014.[261] *The Atlantic* turbocharged the discussion of what it all means when it splashed "The Sex Recession" on the cover of its December 2018 issue. Cover story author Kate Julian focused particularly on the decline in sex among young people, noting, for example, that "in the space of a generation, sex has gone from something most high school students have experienced to something most haven't."[262] She found similar trends in other nations. In Japan, for instance, the percentage of young adults who were virgins increased from about 33 percent to 43 percent in just a decade.

In her article, Julian trotted out an array of possible explanations. They included the usual suspects such as the distractions of smartphones and screens and the awfulness of dating apps, and a few more interesting speculations—for example, perhaps sex is bad or painful more often than we realize. Missing from the lineup was one of the most wide-ranging and consequential possibilities: maybe adults today feel freer to live their most authentic lives, following their true wishes and desires, rather than the dictates of norms and expectations or whatever the popular media is touting. In the realm of sex, that includes resisting the relentless celebration of sex and the pressure to get some, and not just among asexuals.

I love my alone time like no one you've ever met . . . I've been celibate for at least fifteen years. One loses track, because it just doesn't matter— or at least it doesn't matter to me. I have a very romantic relationship with my world every day, and the people who are in it.[263]
—Linda Hamilton, actress

It just doesn't matter; I don't really care; it's not that important. Those are the kinds of accounts I've heard from people who are single at heart. Kristin (fifty-five, Bellingham, Washington) is aromantic. She's not asexual, but sex does not have a big place in her life. She once had a boyfriend, then a husband, and neither was particularly satisfying sexually. Then she had a relationship with a woman. "That was hot," she said. "That was the first time I really felt woken up." In the fifteen years since then, she hasn't had sex. "I don't care. I don't miss it," she said. "I have a great toy box," she added, "and every once in a while, I take out my old battery-powered friends. It's lovely, but not something I feel is necessary at all."

Ed Anderson, who writes the Uncoupled blog, has had hundreds of sexual experiences. About 10 percent were great, another 10 percent were terrible, and all the others were just okay. He no longer thinks sex is worth the effort. When he was young, it was different: sex was very important to him and he thought about it all the time. But at sixty, he said, "It's a relief not to be a puppet on a biological string." He's free to think about other things.[264]

Lucas Bradley is thirty-eight and has never had sex. He is neither asexual nor aromantic. In his blog on Medium, he explains that he has never had sex because he has never pursued sexual relations.

Because sex is a pursuit, it takes time and energy just like any other meaningful pursuit in life. And just because it's sex doesn't mean it gets automatically bumped to the top of the pursuit queue. We live in a fascinating world with an endless array of things to do. All of us, however, only have 168 hours in a week. We need to pick and choose what we pursue.[265]

He has some advice for like-minded souls:

If you, like me, have reached your thirties, forties, and beyond without having sex of any kind, I see you, and I see the power you have. We aren't "virgins." We're diverse people with rich lives and interesting histories.[266]

Joan (seventy-three, Newark, Delaware) has a different reason for abstaining:

I'm unequivocally heterosexual and not asexual. I choose not to act on sexual urges because I'm not willing to take the risks involved in casual sex, and I don't want the rest of the relationship that comes with having monogamous sex.

To Fenton Johnson, author of *At the Center of All Beauty: Solitude and the Creative Life*, voluntary celibacy can be a profound experience:

. . . a conscious decision to refrain from sex can be a powerful incarnation of solitude. Actively inhabited celibacy represents a decision to commit oneself for whatever length of time to a discipline—to forgo one delight (the charms of dalliance, the pleasures of light company) for a different, longer-term undertaking, the deepening of the self.

My monk friends . . . speak with passion of celibacy as a conscious decision to fulfill oneself through love of many rather than of one—a communion with all rather than with a particular individual.[267]

One of the single at heart quiz questions asked, "Think about the possibility that when you go to sleep at night, there might not be anyone else in bed with you. How does that make you feel?" Of those who were clearly single at heart, 94 percent chose the answer, "You are fine with that," compared to just 28 percent of those who were not single at heart.

People who take the single at heart quiz typically choose among the offered responses to each of the questions and leave it at that. But for the question about not having anyone else in bed with you, many of the people who shared their life stories with me could not resist adding their own editorial comments. Those comments included:

- "I actually love it." —Kendra (sixty-nine, San Francisco, California)
- "This is perfect!" —Eva (forty-four, London, England)
- "I love having the bed to myself, although the cats are there." —Beth (fifty-six, San Mateo, California)
- "I am *ecstatic* about that. I hate sharing a bed for sleeping." —Carla (thirty-three, Essex, England)
- "I am great with that." —Anna (fifty-three, Fayetteville, Tennessee)
- "I hog all the covers anyway." —Julie (forty-four, Raleigh, North Carolina)
- "Not just fine with it; I hate having another person in my bed!" —Kristin (fifty-five, Bellingham, Washington)
- "Yippppeeeeee!" —MaryL (sixty-two, Los Angeles, California)

The report that surprised so many people by showing that Americans have been having less sex than they were a few decades ago included another eyebrow-raising finding: The decline was especially steep for people who were married or divorced and much less so, if at all, for lifelong single people. In the early years of the study, married people were having more sex than single people, but by the most recent year, the difference had diminished, and by some ways of looking at the data, may even have reversed.[268] Ordinarily, I love stereotype-defying findings, and this one tells us there is no need to pity people who stay single on the grounds that they are not getting any. But celebrating that is like going along with the premise that having sex is better than not having it, and having lots of sex is better still. I'm much more delighted by the people who skewer the stereotype of poor, lonely single person with no one else in their bed by telling us what they really think of having their bed to themselves: "Yippppeeeeee!"

That's So Aromantic!

I have been in two romantic relationships, both before I considered that I might be aromantic. I've always been rather indifferent toward romance. On both occasions, I got into a romantic relationship with someone I considered a best friend because they had feelings for me, and I didn't want to let them down.
—Jenny, as told to HuffPost[269]

I did not ask about aromanticism on the single at heart quiz, but in the life stories people shared with me, those who are single at heart sometimes described themselves as aromantic, or "aro." Like asexuality, aromanticism also exists on a spectrum.[270] Just as different aces have different attitudes toward sex, so too do different aros have different attitudes toward romance. Some, like Jenny, are indifferent toward it; others are repulsed by it, and still others find the romantic gestures that others covet (teddy bears, slideshows of the couple set to music) to be cheesy and juvenile.

Aromantic, asexual, and single at heart are all overlapping but distinct categories. Some people who are aromantic are also asexual, but others are aromantic but not asexual, and still others are asexual but not aromantic. Similarly, some people who are single at heart are aromantic; others do experience romantic attraction, maybe even intensely, but they still don't want to organize their life around a romantic partner. It's the same for asexuality: on the quiz, 12 percent of the single at heart identified as asexual and that may contribute to their disinterest in building a life around a sexual partner; but the other 88 percent, many of whom may experience quite a lot of sexual attraction, don't want to prioritize a monogamous sexual relationship either.

Because of the relentless pressure to couple up and the rarely challenged belief that coupling is what everyone wants, and because so few people have ever heard of aromanticism, many people get into romantic relationships that don't really interest them; it's what they think they should do. Some even stay in those relationships. It can give them comfort to have the experience, or the appearance of the experience, that everyone is expected to have. But what about the people who have no romantic relationship experience at all?

Romantic Relationship Virgins

In 2017, a story in the *Guardian* broke the internet. It was about a "relationship virgin," a woman who was fifty-four and had never had a boyfriend. She was so ashamed of herself, she would not even use her real name.[271]

Afterward, other relationship virgins shared their stories too. One was Sana Panjwani, twenty-seven, who never had a romantic or sexual relationship. Having grown up in a conservative Desi household in a small town in a Muslim country, she was not too concerned when high school came and went and she had not yet experienced her first love. The subsequent years, though, were more difficult. She felt like she was missing out on an important life experience. She was embarrassed and pretended she really did have a crush. And yet, she said, "I could never bring myself to invite, seek out, or facilitate romance," adding that "the prospect of actually meeting up seemed more stressful than exciting." It was different for other domains of her life: "As a kid, I spent hours dreaming about being a writer—how it would feel to see my name in print, to profile people, to weave stories, and touch readers. Eventually, I became a writer."[272] But she didn't fantasize like that about romantic relationships. "Ultimately, I realized something simple but true: I've never wanted an actual relationship."[273]

Some people who are relationship virgins really and truly want to be in a committed romantic relationship. They experience romantic and sexual attraction and longing, and it can be agonizing when they don't find what they so badly want.

It is different for people like Sana who don't really want a romantic relationship. They probably thought they should want one. Maybe they even wanted to want one. But they just didn't. I think Sana was onto a key sign of how she really felt when she focused on her fantasies. Just as Angela Chen, author of *Ace*, knew what it was like not to think about sex at all when she was alone, Sana did not think much about potential romantic relationships. Not in the way she fantasized about her writing life, imagining how it would unfold and how it would feel.

Sometimes when people seem to be fantasizing about a romantic relationship, what they are really envisioning is the validation. Having something to say when everyone else is going on and on about their crushes. Being seen as experienced. Getting welcomed into the Romantic Couples Club.

When I was a young adult working in my university office, I could sometimes overhear my coupled colleagues making plans to get together on the weekends. I used to wish I could be part of that. What I really wanted, though, was to be included without also having to be coupled.

One of the raps against people who have never had a romantic relationship is that they are not fully adult. Wendy Morris and I documented that harsh judgment in research we conducted.[274] But I don't think I was ever less adult than when I was in the dating game, trying to be someone I was not. I was only a passive participant, saying yes when asked, but still. I should have taken the big fat hints that romantic coupling just didn't interest me. Like that time in college when a date asked me which of two movies I wanted to see, and I chose the one that started fifteen minutes later so I could have fifteen more minutes to myself.

Choosing a life that is not built around a romantic relationship is about more than those snippets of time you will never get back. It is about the joys and the psychological richness of living your most meaningful and fulfilling life. It is about choosing authenticity, even if your authentic path is not the most validated or valued one. There is nothing more adult than that.

Today's happy romantic relationship virgins understand that single life offers a world of possibilities. Here's what Mollie told *Glamour UK*: "Not looking for love has led me to so much more than I ever thought—a carefree happiness that isn't dictated by somebody else; a motivation to give myself a life full of beautiful things; a gratitude toward the life I'm carving out for myself; and a solitude that I bask in."[275]

Acadia (thirty-six, Melbourne, Australia) has never been on an official date. She's never felt romantically or sexually attracted to anyone. Rather than feeling ashamed, she is proud of how psychologically rich her life has been:

> Technically I am a relationship virgin, but I don't think of myself that way. That title feels like I am inexperienced. I feel I have experienced so much more of life than I *ever* would have if I was partnered. All the places I've gone, the people I've met, the shows I've been in, the friends I've made, the work I'm so proud of doing . . . I just feel so *blessed* that I've been able to live my life freely.

Acadia's perspective is mature and wise. Let's follow her lead. What if, instead of putting romantic relationship experience on a pedestal, we instead valued and celebrated all the accomplishments and experiences that bring us joy? Why shouldn't we feel equally proud, or even more proud, of having lifelong friends? Of feeling comfortable in solitude, for hours or even days on end? Of caring passionately about something or someone other than a romantic partner? Of living authentically? Of making a difference in the world?

The Secret Strengths of Young People Who Are Not Preoccupied with Romantic Relationships

I definitely remember from my days in an all-boys' secondary school (between the ages of eleven and eighteen) that I was always an odd one out in terms of being interested, or indeed in my case *not* being interested, in pairing up with the opposite sex or indeed not being particularly impressed with gawping at pictures of the latest attractive model du jour.

—Steve (thirty-nine, Bolton, England)

When Brooke Douglas was a graduate student at the University of Georgia, she read dozens of articles by social scientists about adolescent romantic relationships. She noticed certain assumptions in those articles—for example, that adolescent romantic relationships are important for personal development and psychological health. That made her wonder: is there something wrong with teens who don't date? When she and a colleague analyzed data from nearly six hundred tenth graders, they found just the opposite. The students who had never dated (or maybe had had just one date) were less depressed than their peers who did date. When the teachers were asked to evaluate the students, without ever being told which ones had dated, their assessments were the same—they saw the students who did not date as less depressed than the students who did. They also saw them as more socially skilled and as having superior leadership abilities.[276]

Follow adolescents over time, as they get involved in romantic relationships or don't, and you can see the unfolding of feelings of depression. In a study of a nationally representative sample of more than eight thousand adolescents, ages twelve through seventeen, feelings of depression increased over the course of a year to a greater extent for the teens who became romantically involved than for those who did not. That's not because the daters broke up; even the teens who stayed in the same relationship the whole time became more depressed.[277] Romantic relationships were especially depressing for adolescents who were not particularly attracted to people of any gender, but still got into a romantic relationship.[278]

The teens who got romantically involved also began drinking more than those who did not, and they engaged in more troubling behaviors such as getting into fights. The boys suffered academically—their grades slipped—and the girls lost out interpersonally—their relationships with their parents became more difficult.

It doesn't get better with age or romantic relationship experience. That's what Professor Matthew D. Johnson and his colleagues discovered when they studied 554 Germans who, over the course of a multiyear study, had two romantic relationships. The oldest were forty-one when they were questioned for the first time. Just as the other researchers had found in their study of adolescents, Professor Johnson and his colleagues discovered that people felt worse as their romantic relationships progressed—they were more depressed and less satisfied with their lives, and their self-esteem took a hit too.[279]

It wasn't all bad. The participants felt good at the start of their second romantic relationship—they were less depressed and more satisfied with themselves and their lives than they were before that relationship started. But it didn't last. Soon, the usual trajectory resumed—they started feeling worse about themselves and their lives. Long-term studies of marriage often show the same pattern: around the time of the wedding, people who stay married feel a brief frisson of happiness. That dissipates over time, and they end up no happier than they were when they were single. People who eventually divorce typically do not experience that brief uptick in happiness around the time of the wedding, and they end up less happy than when they were single.[280]

At the beginning of the study of the teens who did or did not date, the students were asked a key question: to what extent were they hoping to become romantically involved in the coming year? The teens who were wishing for romance were especially likely to become depressed over time, regardless of whether or not their wish came true. The teens who said they were not interested in becoming romantically involved that year (an early sign of being single at heart?) did better.[281]

The same psychological dynamics continue into young adulthood. In a study of people ages eighteen to twenty-nine, those who were not in a romantic relationship and did not care all that much about being in one were doing better than those who were not in a relationship but really wanted to be. They were less depressed and less lonely. They were also no more depressed than their peers who were in a romantic relationship. The young adults who were romantically involved, though, were more satisfied with their lives than either group of uninvolved peers. What they had done had likely brought them admiration and respect—they were in the Couples Club. The accomplishments of the uncoupled had probably gone unrecognized.[282]

Suppose the uncoupled were particularly skilled at friendship, which is likely to be especially true of people who are single at heart. For twenty-year-olds, will that matter as much to their success a decade later as their romantic relationship experience? In an intensive, decades-long study, 205 Minnesotans were interviewed in person and their parents and clinical psychologists were consulted too. The participants who had a close, confiding friendship when they were twenty were doing especially well ten years later. They were succeeding at work, and they were more likely to have a close friendship than their peers who had no such friendship when they were twenty. They were more likely to have a close relationship with a romantic partner too. In contrast, romantic experience at age twenty had no relevance to future success. The young adults who, at twenty, had been in a close romantic relationship for more than a brief period, were no more likely to be successful at work or with friends—and they were not even any more likely to have a close romantic relationship.[283]

Steve (quoted at the beginning of this section) thought of himself as the odd person out when, as a teen, he did not share his peers' interest in romantic pursuits. If a hoard of developmental psychologists had descended upon him, maybe some of them would have been concerned. But as Brooke Douglas learned when she put those kinds of assumptions to the test, teens who do not date often do better than those who do. Steve was thirty-nine when he shared his life story, and he still had not been on a date. Like so many others who are single at heart, he is living his most authentic life, a psychologically rich life full of travel, adventures, and work that he loves. He is living happily ever after.

Our Sensuous Lives

> I inhaled the aroma of rotisserie chicken dripping
> on roasted fingerling potatoes.
> —Marie (forty-six, Northern California),
> describing a time when she was in Paris

During the worst of COVID, I was super careful. I kept my distance from other humans and did not even do my own grocery shopping. Even after the threat seemed to have subsided a bit, I stayed cautious. I knew that COVID could be utterly miserable, even deadly, and that at my age, my risk was amplified. But even if I could dodge the most menacing symptoms, there was one I could not fathom enduring: the loss of taste. I love good food. I fantasize about it every single day. Delicious food, beautifully presented, makes me very happy. I don't understand all those online articles explaining how to get rid of the smell of food after you've cooked; I adore having those scents wafting through my home.

If I wake up the next day, and the faint whiffs of last night's dinner linger in the air, I start my day smiling.

Based on the stories shared with me, my guess is that people who are single at heart, regardless of our sexual or romantic orientations or attractions, are especially likely to value sensuous experiences. I think that's akin to our inclination to be savorers, that I discussed in the chapter on solitude. Tastes, smells, sights, sounds, feelings, and sensations that bring us joy are all examples of the sensuality of our lives. When I asked Eva (forty-four, London, England) what makes her happy, she unfurled a long list, a compendium of sensuousness. The items included "an early walk in the park watching a glorious sunrise, feeling the fresh breeze on my cheeks" and "fresh sheets after a nice bath with oils and salts!"

For Craig (forty-one, Newport News, Virginia) it is the sound of music that is rapturous—especially at concerts. He has been going to concerts, thinking about concerts, and for the past few years, he has blogged about every concert he has attended. "Concerts are my medicine," he said. "When I'm dancing at a show, all my issues just disappear and I'm in the moment."

Physicality can feel sensuous and empowering. Here's what Catherine Clifford, an ultramarathon runner, shared in her essay, "On Running and Asexual Embodiment":

> I've been a runner for over twenty years, and as such, I think of my body as the body of a runner. When I run, my legs and lungs immediately return to the rhythms and motions of familiar corporeal ritual. In running I exist as something at once more powerful and more knowing.[284]

Touch can be one of the most powerful sensuous experiences, and there are so many kinds of touching beyond the sexual. I'm a hugger. I love to greet friends and relatives with big hugs, or at least the ones who are not touch-averse. In *Friends: Understanding the Power of Our Most Important Relationships*,

Robin Dunbar suggests that we don't always recognize just how delightful all that hugging and patting and all the other forms of physical contact we have with our friends can be. All sorts of other sensuous experiences we share with our friends, such as "laughter, singing and dancing, storytelling and feasting," can also bring their own natural highs, he noted.[285]

Eva enjoys the tactile pleasures of massages. During COVID, Ketaki (thirty-four, Manipal, India) missed human touch. She was injured near the onset of the pandemic and was grateful for the touch that was part of her physiotherapy. No one I interviewed mentioned cuddle parties—safe places to enjoy affectionate, nonsexual touching and cuddling—but in post-pandemic times, I expect to hear more about them.

> My two dogs let me know when the mail has arrived and are pretty good at keeping my feet warm in the winter. Snuggling with them makes me happy. —Sonya (forty-seven, Parkersburg, West Virginia)

Touch sometimes comes all wrapped up with other sensuous treats. Our pets, for example, can be warm, purring, cuddly, and adorable bundles of joy. Iris (sixty-five, Portugal) cuddles with her ten-year-old cat in front of CNN and Netflix. Babies can be like that too. Maria (fifty-two, Beverly, Massachusetts) has a suggestion for people who are looking for more nonsexual touching than they are getting: volunteer at the local hospital to hold babies in the NICU.

People who derive great pleasure from sensuality, and not just the sensuality that is part of sexual experiences, have easy and nearly limitless access to joy. No one needs privacy, or any kind of partner, to look out a well-placed window, or to soak in the view over and over and over again. Food lovers get to indulge that sensuality multiple times a day, every single day. Craig never tires of music. Sonya's dogs never get boring or annoying; they are perpetual happiness generators. Catherine, who has been running outrageously long distances for decades, sometimes through forests, still reaps "the blessings of the woods" every single time. When the single at heart create homes that are sensual sanctuaries, we get to bask in the comforts we have curated every moment of every day that we spend there.

Flipping the Script

"Losing at Love? A Coach May Help."[286]
—Headline in the *New York Times*

In a blog post, "'Losing at Love?' You're Playing the Wrong Game," Lucas Bradley pointed out that the readers of the *Times* article were losing out at dating and romantic relationships, not love in its most generous, expansive forms. He said that he preferred to count the ways he is winning at love, and listed ten examples, such as:

- When the creative work of another person moves me to tears, I'm winning at love.
- When my cat greets me and purrs on my arrival home, I'm winning at love.
- When I see someone I haven't spoken to in weeks or months and the conversation picks up like it was yesterday, I'm winning at love.
- When I see how relationships grow organically with others in my life without the need to force things to be a certain way, I'm winning at love.
- When I embrace the totality of my life experience and understand that none of it needs to be served up to others for judgment of my worthiness, I'm winning at love.

Our Intimate Lives

I am often overwhelmed by how much love is in my life, from my friends, my family, and the animals I am so lucky to know. I think a lot of people think that if you don't have romantic love, you're missing something, but having had it in the past, I can safely say I feel that I have more love in my life now than when I was coupled.

—Carla (thirty-three, Essex, England)

For the single at heart, love is inclusive and unfettered. We don't try to confine love or intimacy to romantic partners, nor do we place such partners atop a hierarchy. We decide for ourselves whom to love and whose love matters most to us, and as Carla indicated by mentioning animals, our love lives aren't just about humans.

My family and many friends love me, and I feel their love every day even if we don't talk. My cat lets me know he loves me every time I walk in the door. My church family is like my second family. —Julie (forty-four, Raleigh, North Carolina)

Many people who are single at heart live alone. That doesn't mean that love isn't with us all the time, as Julie revealed when she said that she feels the love of her family and friends every day. The love we experienced earlier in our lives can endure too, as Joan (seventy-three, Newark, Delaware) noted when she said, "I was deeply loved growing up, and I think that's something that stays with me as part of who I am, just as a sense of community stays with me even if none of my friends is physically present."

I previously described the many kinds of humans, nonhumans, and meaningful entities who are part of our social convoys. So too are they part of our love lives. On the "On Being" podcast, Sandra Cisneros, author of *The House on Mango Street*, put it this way: "I feel very loved by the universe and the trees and the clouds and the sky and the sunsets and my dogs and the people who are in my life and my students."[287]

When enumerating the sources and objects of their love, Daz (thirty-eight, Northern England) mentioned art; Sonya (forty-seven, Parkersburg, West Virginia) pointed to her creative endeavors; Mary (thirty-three, Buffalo, New York) and Ketaki (thirty-four, Manipal, India) mentioned plants and flowers and nature; and Andrea (twenty-nine, New York City) said she loves her experiences and memories. All of them also named people they loved and who loved them, but they didn't stop at that obvious category.

The single at heart understand intimacy as a much more expansive experience than just sexual or romantic closeness. Liz (sixty, Washington, DC) said, "When people share their deepest sorrows, fears, and joys with you, that's intimacy." Marie (forty-six, Northern California) said, "Meetings of the mind register as intimate to me. That seems easiest when any sexual dynamic is removed. I bond with friends in profound connection." The last word goes to Kristin (fifty-five, Bellingham, Washington) who shared: "When my friend Beth's dad was dying, I remember holding her in my arms while she cried, for the longest time. If that's not intimacy, I don't know what is."

Advice For the Single at Heart

Your view of intimacy is probably already much broader, more inclusive, and less judgmental than many other people's views are. You know that all sorts of sexual and romantic preferences are just fine, including having no interest at all. You understand that love and intimacy are much bigger than just romantic love or sexual intimacy. You know that an appreciation of sensuousness can be especially fulfilling, and it is something you can enjoy just about every moment of every day. What you get to do now, if you want to, is to be a model for others. There is so much that others can learn from you.

At the same time, you don't owe anyone a report on your sex life, romantic interests, or lack of interests. If you do want to talk about any of it, do so unapologetically. When you describe in a matter of fact or enthusiastic way your asexuality, aromanticism, kinks, solo sex, unbundling of sex from romance or monogamy, or anything else that interests you but may dismay others, you normalize it for everyone else. You become a shame-repellant. That's powerful and important.

For Our Allies

Don't ask about our sex lives or expect us to entertain you with stories from dating adventures. Feel free to ask us about the people we care about and who care about us; that's a great way to show that you too understand that love and intimacy come in many flavors, and it gives us an opening to talk about sexual intimacy if we want to.

If you are an educator, you can take the lead in introducing and normalizing all different ways of experiencing intimacy beyond just the sexual. You can inoculate people who don't date or who have never had a romantic relationship from feeling shamed and dissuade those who may be tempted to do the shaming. If you are a mental health professional, keep up with the evolving thinking and research on experiences such as asexuality, aromanticism, and solo polyamory, so you can be more attuned to what your clients really are feeling or desiring, even if they do not have the vocabulary to describe it or feel shamed about what they want or don't want.

For People Who Are Intrigued by Single Life, But Have Concerns

If you are not all that interested in sex or romance, living single is your chance to claim the life that suits you best. If you have sexual or romantic preferences that are considered unusual, living single is your chance to explore them without risking the disapproval of a conventional romantic partner. You get to design your own intimacy map, and you get to reconfigure that map if or when you want to incorporate something new. If you are drawn to single life but worry about missing out on the sex and intimacy that a conventional romantic partner might offer, be clear-eyed about the latter. Having a romantic partner under the same roof is no guarantee that the two of you will always want the same kinds and amounts of intimacy at the same time, or that neither of you will ever be tempted to stray. And the research shows that single people who are not that interested in unsingling themselves are about as sexually satisfied as married people.

8

How Life Turns Out

At every phase in your life, look at your options.
Please, do not select the boring ones.[288]
—Barbara Hillary

That was the advice Barbara Hillary offered in the commencement
address she gave at The New School in New York in 2017. Hillary was a
lifelong single person with no children, and she never chose boring.

When she learned that no black woman had ever made it to the North
Pole, she resolved to be the first. To get there, she would be dropped off by
helicopter in Norway. Getting the rest of the way, another thirty miles, would
require up to ten hours a day of cross-country skiing. The problem? She had
never skied before. "It wasn't a popular sport in Harlem," she deadpanned.[289]
She hired a personal trainer, took skiing lessons, lifted weights, and worked
out on a treadmill.

Reaching the top of the world was exhilarating. "I have never experienced
such sheer joy and excitement," she said. "I was screaming, jumping up and
down."[290] She was seventy-five.

Old age is supposedly when we lifelong single people get our
comeuppance. Sure, we get to have our independence and our adventures
and maybe even some happiness as young single people, but how happy will
we be when our youth and energy are behind us? What will happen when we
fall ill and there is no one there to help us?

Hillary faced serious illness long before she grew old. She had breast
cancer in her twenties. Then, at sixty-seven, it was lung cancer. Surgery cost

her a quarter of her breathing capacity. Undeterred, she headed to Quebec for some dogsledding and to Manitoba to photograph polar bears. Then the North Pole.

She wasn't finished. At seventy-nine, she trekked to the South Pole. There, she savored "the joy of silence."[291] When she was eighty-seven, she visited Outer Mongolia. Contacted by a reporter from the *New Yorker* a few months before her death at eighty-eight, she was planning her next trip, to Russia.[292]

Hillary's travels started out as adventures but along the way, she was struck by the devastating impact of climate change on places she came to love. She lectured on the topic and arranged future excursions to learn even more.

Hillary had a big, expansive, generous life even before her travels. She earned bachelor's and master's degrees in gerontology, worked as a nurse, drove a taxi, founded a neighborhood association and a magazine. She grew tomatoes and roses, and, according to a friend, liked "archery, guns and knives, big trucks and big dogs."[293] She celebrated her birthdays by giving gifts to the people who had been especially kind to her that year.

Hillary grew up poor, but "there was no such thing as woe is me," she told The New School graduates.[294] When she set out to conquer the North Pole, she had nowhere near the money she needed. That was before the days of GoFundMe and Kickstarter, so she sent letters. One went to then mayor of New York, Michael Bloomberg, who relayed her inquiry to the Department for the Aging, who in turn sent her a letter describing the activities available at the senior center. "If I'm going to the North Pole, why the hell do I need a senior center?" she asked.[295]

Hillary was utterly unapologetic about her lifelong singlehood. When told that she looked youthful, she credited her singleness. She didn't feign interest in coupling to try to fit in and she did not want to spend a lot of time with those who were preoccupied with such matters. She and two of her friends who traveled domestically called themselves "By Invitation Only."

"We don't want to hear about your miserable marriage, your boyfriend. You wanna talk about polar bears and the state of the world? You're in," she told the *New Yorker*.[296]

Not having a romantic partner did not limit Hillary's life in her youth or in her older years, it swung open the doors to both ends of the earth. She lived the ultimate single at heart life—joyful, authentic, and psychologically rich. She flipped the script of conventional adult life and redefined what it meant to live a good and meaningful life. Rather than settling into an insular domestic life and leaning on a spouse to cover half or fewer of the tasks of everyday life, rather than folding herself into a smaller life as she aged, Hillary kept learning new skills and mastering formidable feats, for better or for worse, through sickness and health, until death parted her from the earth.

Barbara Hillary was, of course, an exceptional individual. But in living a life that just seemed to get bigger and better over time, even into old age, she may have been typical of people who are single at heart. Old age is supposed to be particularly frightening to people who arrive there without a committed romantic partner, but the single at heart are writing a different story. For us, old age is when we reap the rewards of our long and loving embrace of single life.

Aging While Single: Why It Just Keeps Getting Better

The great gift of aging is the ability to release yourself from responsibility for others' reaction to you. The relinquishing of such burden comes with an additional prize: finding people's disapproval or shock about who you are ridiculous.[297]
—Keturah Kendrick, *No Thanks: Black, Female, and Living in the Martyr-Free Zone*

Despite all the scaremongering about being old and single and supposedly alone—scaremongering aimed with special intensity at single women—single life, in some important ways, just keeps getting better and better with age. And not just for people who are single at heart. There are more fellow solo singles in later life than there were when we were younger.[298] As we age, fewer and fewer single people even want a partner.[299] There's less pressure too.[300] Those annoying relatives who kept asking if there is anyone special in our life have mostly zipped it. What's more, we no longer care what they think, if we ever did. Add that all up and the result is great satisfaction: as we age, single people just keep getting more and more satisfied with their lives, for the four reasons I just previewed.[301]

First, our numbers. Consider the results of a Pew Research Center report, based on a nationally representative sample of US adults in 2019, that focused specifically on solo singles—they were not married, not cohabiting, and they were not in a committed romantic relationship.[302] Overall, 31 percent of Americans who were eighteen and older were solo singles. Age, though, mattered a lot. Among women in their thirties and forties, only 19 percent were solo singles, the lowest of any age group. But look what happens by the time they reach sixty-five and beyond—nearly half (49 percent) are solo singles! In later life, if you don't have a spouse or a serious romantic partner, you are no longer the outlier—you are practically the norm. (It is different for men. The percentage of solo singles decreases with age, from 51 percent for the youngest group, to 27 percent all through the thirties, forties, fifties, and early sixties, and then down to 21 percent for those sixty-five and older.)

Second, our desires. Studies of more than thirty-three hundred Dutch adults without romantic partners showed that all across their adult lives, from ages eighteen through seventy-five, the desire to have a partner kept declining.[303] Tap into just about any random study and you will find the same thing. Take, for example, that 2019 Pew survey.[304] Across all ages, half of all solo single people said they were not interested in a committed romantic relationship or even a date. The youngest adults (eighteen to twenty-nine) were the most interested: 63 percent wanted a committed relationship or at least a date. But for the solo singles sixty-five and older, only 22 percent were interested in any of that.

Jane Gross, who founded "The New Old Age" blog for the *New York Times*, has never married. Throughout her twenties and thirties, she said, "all I wanted was joined-at-the-hip, happily-ever-after togetherness, with babies, even a mother-in-law."[305] By sixty-five, though, she felt differently and considers herself single at heart: "I know that I'm greedy for the quiet of my own home at the end of a long day. And I'm grateful not to have to sit through movies I don't want to see, stay at parties longer than necessary, eat at 'proper' meal times, collect towels from the floor, or have someone follow me from room to room, expecting me to talk when I don't feel like talking."[306]

Third, the pressures. The Pew researchers asked the solo single people how much pressure they felt from friends, family members, and society to be in a committed romantic relationship. All three sources of pressure subsided with age.[307] About half of the youngest adults (eighteen to twenty-nine) felt some or a lot of pressure from family members and society to unsingle themselves; for the oldest adults, though (sixty-five and older), only about 20 percent felt pressured. With age, friends became less annoying, but they were less annoying to begin with; even among the youngest group, only 28 percent said they felt pressured by their friends to abandon their single lives. The oldest solo singles are the most blissfully free. More than half of those who are sixty-five and older say they feel no pressure at all from friends, family, or society.

Fourth, the satisfaction. Studies of adults who do not have a romantic partner show that once they get to their forties and beyond, they just keep getting more and more satisfied with their single lives. One set of researchers discovered that when they studied German singles,[308] and another set found the same thing when they studied Dutch singles.[309] People who stay single also become more confident about who they really are. A study of US adults at midlife compared, over a five-year period, more than one thousand people who had always been single to more than three thousand who were continuously married.[310] It was the single people who were more likely to agree with statements such as, "I judge myself by what I think is important, not by the values of what others think is important" and "I have confidence in my opinions, even if they are different from the way most other people think."

As good as it can get for all solo singles, it gets even better for the single at heart. We've got this. We've been preparing for it for as long as we understood ourselves as single at heart and committed ourselves to the life we love the most.

Flipping the Script

"Perhaps it is only after midlife (around forty) when the peak period of partnering opportunities has passed for both genders, single individuals come to terms with being single and becoming better at finding ways to be happy with single life the older they get."[311]
—Yoobin Park, Elizabeth Page-Gould, and Geoff MacDonald,
"Satisfying Singlehood as a Function of Age and Cohort"

The social scientists are trying to explain their findings that single people between forty and eighty become more and more satisfied with their single lives as they grow older. Imagine if they had found the same thing for married people (they didn't) and said this: "Perhaps it is only after midlife (around forty) when the peak period of opportunities for having affairs has passed for both genders, married individuals come to terms with being married and becoming better at finding ways to be happy with married life the older they get."

More Joyful, More Psychologically Rich, More Authentic

The longer I'm single, the more I love it. I can't imagine life any other way.
—Sonya (forty-seven, Parkersburg, West Virginia)

For just about everyone who is single at heart, single life just gets better and better over time. Those hallmarks of the single at heart life—joyfulness, psychological richness, and authenticity—become even more deeply experienced. Marie (forty-six, Northern California) nodded to the joyfulness when she said that her single life "just gets sweeter." MaryL (Los Angeles), said, "I'm sixty-two and life is *so* good it scares me at times!"

Throughout our adult lives we pursued the interests and passions that made our lives so rich psychologically and so consistent with who we really are. With no romantic partner at the center of our lives, we did not need to bend or deny our wishes or plans to accommodate a partner. Because we were not marking time, waiting and hoping for such a partner to appear, we did not put off living our single lives as fully and completely as our opportunities and resources would allow. We continued to learn and grow. In the midlife study that compared lifelong single people to continuously married people over a five-year period, it was the single people who were especially likely to agree with statements such as "I think it is important to have new experiences that challenge how you think about yourself and the world."[312]

In later life we continue to get to be the deciders. If, for example, we want to keep working into our old age even if we don't need the money, we do. In contrast, married people's decisions are often influenced by whether their spouse wants them to keep working, research shows.[313]

Some of us had to struggle to get to the point of recognizing and embracing our true single at heart selves, as I've already discussed. The social pressures that push us all to couple up, and to believe that coupled life is the natural, normal, and superior life, are relentless. There's a lot to overcome. In our thirties, if we had friends and relatives who were already marching down the conventional coupled path, or parents who were making their coupling wishes known to us even more insistently, some of us may have found it especially challenging to stand our ground and refuse to let the seeds of self-doubt implant themselves in our souls. Once we got past our thirties and sailed into midlife, that's when we got to live even more confidently and authentically, and when our single lives just kept getting better and better.

Carla (Essex, England) was just thirty-three when she first shared her life story with me, but she already had a wise insight into the psychological dynamics of aging while single. "My actual experience of living single hasn't changed that much," she said. "It's always been good and I've always preferred living alone to living with other people. My *perception* of living single has changed hugely for the better, based mostly on listening to how I actually feel about it rather than how I am supposed to view it. I can't see myself changing it, now. Aside from my grief over Dad, in the rest of my life I am the happiest I've ever been."

Getting to live authentically may be one of the most profound rewards of embracing our single lives. Ginny (fifty-nine, Ontario, Canada) said, "As time passes, I feel as though I'm becoming more myself. I'm expressing opinions I would never dared have expressed before, accepting feelings that were quashed before, setting limits to human interactions that drain me." Peggy (sixty-seven, Atlanta, Georgia) said, "I am more secure and know more who I am every day."

We Invested in Ourselves

I began retirement planning in my thirties because I was the only one
who was going to do it. I can only count on my own income.
I have set and met financial goals, found a house to purchase
so I can age in place, and keep on top of retirement accounts.
I feel very secure in my planning for old age.
—Sonya (forty-seven, Parkersburg, West Virginia)

Stereotypically, people in Barbara Hillary's demographic have five strikes against them—they are older, they are women, they do not have a spouse, they don't have kids, and they are black. They are presumed to be in poor health, physically and emotionally, a social burden and a drain on medical services. A professor of social work, Julie Cwikel, wanted to know if any of that was true.[314] She and her colleagues addressed the first four of those presumed obstacles, analyzing data from more than ten thousand Australian women in their seventies. They compared the lifelong single women who had no kids to married women with and without kids, and previously married women with and without kids.

They found that in later life, the lifelong single women were not just keeping up with the other women but surpassing them in many ways. They were the most optimistic and the least stressed. They had larger social networks than the married women. They were more likely to be active members of formal social groups. They were strikingly healthier: they had the fewest number of diagnoses of major illnesses and the healthiest body mass index; they were least likely to be smokers and most likely to be nondrinkers. They were not a burden on the health care system when they did need care, as they were most likely to have their own private health insurance. They weren't burdening their families either. They were no more likely to be cared for by family members than any of the other women. The researchers concluded that, far from being a "problem" group, "their life experiences and opportunities had prepared them for a successful and productive older age."

In the United States too, lifelong single people, when they get to their later years, are often doing better than their peers who invested in marriage. Social scientists sat down with 530 people age sixty-five and older who were divorced or widowed or had always been single.[315] They interviewed men as well as women, and they deliberately recruited just as many blacks as whites. They asked the participants about the strains in their lives. Was there anyone to take care of them if they needed help? Did they have anyone with whom they could share their everyday life experiences? Was it getting more difficult to have an active social life? Did they have the intimacy they would like? Did the future look more difficult to them?

As in the Australian study, it was the lifelong single people who reported the least strain. In the US study, that was especially true for the lifelong singles who were black. The previously married seniors were the ones who were less likely to have the help that they needed, or the social life or the intimacy that they wanted. It was those divorced and widowed people, more so than the lifelong single people, who didn't have anyone with whom to share their day-to-day experiences and who were less optimistic about the future. In a study of Dutch seniors, those who had always been single were also more satisfied with their lives than those who were divorced or widowed.[316]

Maybe for the previously married seniors, single life came as a shock. Perhaps they thought that, having found a partner, they had old age covered. They had that Magical Mythical Romantic Partner. Their spouse would be there to grow old with them and to care for them. The single at heart have a whole different perspective. Once we embraced our true single at heart selves, we didn't count on a real or imagined future spouse to be our caretakers, fixers, or financial backstops. Instead we invested in ourselves, we invested in The Ones (instead of The One), and we prepared for a single life that would last for life.

Embracing our single at heart selves and investing in our single lives are what matters most. Some people who are single at heart were previously married. Some tried to put a romantic partner at the center of their lives over and over again, until they realized they were chasing someone else's version of the good life, not their own. It is never too late to understand who you really are, and then reap the rewards of living accordingly.

Optimism: that's the theme that pops up again and again. In the Australian study, it was the lifelong single women in their seventies, with no kids, who were the most optimistic. In the US study, it was the lifelong single men and women who were the least likely to say that the future looked difficult to them. The American Association of Retired Persons (AARP) also found evidence for the optimism of "solo agers," people older than fifty who live alone, are not married or in a long-term partnered relationship, and have no living children.[317] Those solo agers were about as likely as the other adults in their age group to feel very or extremely optimistic about their quality of life as they grew older, and they were a bit less likely to feel pessimistic. Only 13 percent said they felt sad.

It is remarkable that all those groups are so optimistic. The lifelong single people in the first two studies never did do what the prevailing ideologies and mythologies told them they were supposed to do—find The One and create a life centered around that person. That's what was presented to them as the ticket to happiness and the truest, deepest source of confidence and optimism. In the Australian study, the lifelong single people also did not have that other much-touted source of meaning and presumed reason to care about the future—they didn't have kids. The solo agers surveyed by AARP may or may not have had a spouse or romantic partner in the past, but now they had no partner, no kids, and they were living alone. They were even once condescendingly and misleadingly called "elder orphans."

The writers of the deficit narratives of single life look at all those people and expect to find them wallowing in self-pity. Instead they are confident and optimistic. What's more, their optimism serves them especially well. In *Happy Singlehood*, Elyakim Kislev reported that both married and unmarried people were happier when they were more optimistic. But the link was even stronger for the single people. They got even more happiness out of their optimism than the married people did.[318]

For the single at heart in particular, our optimism is powerful because it is earned. In defiance of a lifetime of being told that our lives just didn't measure up to the lives of coupled people, we persisted. We were warned that we couldn't do it, but we did it. We built joyful, psychologically rich, and authentic lives of our own.

We Invested in "The Ones"

Those who had limited their social interaction to the spouse or partner
often fail to become reintegrated when the relationship had ended.[319]
—Jan Eckhard, sociologist, "Social isolation as a consequence of
transitions in partner relationships"

The single at heart don't get involved romantically with another person, put
that person at the center of their lives, and demote their friends. We continue
to value our friends and we are more likely than people who are not single at
heart to welcome more friends into our lives and not marginalize the friends
we already have. As we get older, those of us who have never married are
also spared another potential friend-winnowing experience: We don't lose
custody of any friends after a divorce, as, for example, when some friends
side with an ex.

Becoming a widow has the potential to be even more isolating than
getting divorced, particularly in later life. In Heidelberg University sociologist
Jan Eckhard's study of nearly thirty-one thousand relationship endings
among German adults, Eckhard found that younger people who experienced
divorces or other breakups of romantic relationships sometimes become
socially isolated for a few years, but many eventually rebuild social networks.[320]
It is harder for older people whose spouse has died. The extreme examples
are the 9 percent of people who are married or living with a romantic partner
and have no other social contact at all—not with friends and not with family,
and they don't participate in any clubs or civic organizations. They were the
most likely to be isolated and stay isolated after their partner died. Maybe
they took those love song lyrics a bit too seriously, as they looked at their
spouse and thought, *You are my everything.* Then when their spouse died, they
had no one.

Bronnie Ware, an Australian nurse who spent years working in palliative
care, heard many epiphanies of people who were dying. She described them

in her internationally best-selling book, *The Top Five Regrets of the Dying*.[321] The fourth most common regret was, "I wish I had stayed in touch with my friends." The single at heart are more likely to stay connected with their friends and so less likely to die with that regret. (I'll get to the number one regret later.)

Over the course of our adult lives, people who are single—and especially the single at heart—stand out for our embrace of The Ones rather than just The One. We typically have more friends, we invest more in our friends, and we get more out of our friendships. We think about the people who matter to us in more expansive ways. "Relationship," to us, does not just mean a romantic relationship; we have relationships with lots of different kinds of people. And family is not just about the people to whom we are related by blood, marriage, or adoption. We decide who counts as family.

As we age, all of these psychological dynamics remain just as significant, or they become even more so. The study of the significance of friendship in ninety-nine nations that I mentioned previously showed that the people who valued their friends were especially likely to be happy, healthy, and satisfied with their lives.[322] It also showed that that valuing of friendship seemed to be even more of a boon to the happiness, health, and life satisfaction of older people than younger ones.

But friends are too often regarded as "just friends," people who just aren't that important in the big scheme of things. According to the stories we've been told our whole lives, no one is supposed to be better for our psychological health than a spouse. As we age, a spouse is supposed to be the person who protects us most effectively from feeling lonely, depressed, or stressed. Anyone who does not have a spouse would do well to have someone as similar as possible to a spouse, we are told. There's a hierarchy of four categories. Older people who live with a romantic partner who is not a spouse will not do as well as the married people, but they will do better than single people who are dating, who in turn will do better than single people who do not have any kind of romantic partner. But is that true?

Matthew Wright and Susan Brown of Bowling Green University put the conventional wisdom to the test.[323] In their representative national sample of US adults aged between fifty-seven and eighty-five, they found no significant differences whatsoever among the women in the four categories. Their position in the romantic partnership hierarchy had nothing to do with how lonely, depressed, or stressed they were. For the men, having a romantic partner mattered more than it did for the women. For example, the cohabiting men were less likely to be depressed or lonely than either category of single men. But the men who were dating did not do any better in any way than the single men, and the married men were actually more depressed than the cohabiting men.

What did matter, for both the women and the men, was straightforward: having supportive friends and family. The women and men who had friends or relatives they could confide in, people they could turn to when they had a problem, were the ones who were most likely to be protected from depression or stress. The women with supportive friends or relatives were also protected from feeling lonely.

In a study of twenty-three hundred American adults ages sixty-two and older by Ashley E. Ermer and Christine M. Proulx, the researchers found that seniors who had more confidants and people they could turn to when they needed help were less likely to feel depressed or lonely, and they were happier too.[324] Having that social support was beneficial to all of the older people, regardless of whether they had a romantic partner. In important ways, though, the older single people were doing even better than the older coupled people. They named more people who were there for them as confidants or helpers. They were emotionally closer to those people. Compared to people with romantic partners, they saw their family members as more likely to be there for them, and they had more interactions with their neighbors. Perhaps most importantly, the single seniors benefited even more from the important people in their lives. Having confidants and potential helpers protected them from depression and loneliness even more than it protected coupled people, and it was linked to greater happiness too.

For some single people, no one is more important to them than their relatives. Brandy Renee McCann and Katherine R. Allen learned that when they talked at great length with the kinds of single women who are often neglected by researchers, the rural poor.[325] The fourteen women in their study were all working class seniors, ages fifty-two to seventy-two, who were born in rural Appalachia and still lived there. They described themselves as evangelical Christians or as "believers." Some were separated, divorced, or widowed, and others had always been single. A few lived with grown children who were financially dependent on them and two were caring for their parents and lived with them; the others lived alone. They may have been single and living alone, but nearly all of them were living on family land and surrounded by family. The homes of immediate and extended family members were often just steps away.

Family was a part of their everyday lives, and for most of them, it always had been. They grew up together, they worshipped together, and now, in later life, they were there for one another. The single women who did not have children had close relationships with their nieces and nephews. Nine of the fourteen women had no interest in romantic relationships; they were the ones whose lives were most interconnected with the lives of their nearby relatives and who felt most fulfilled by their families. For them, becoming coupled "would disrupt family life," McCann and Allen noted.[326] Putting a romantic partner at the center of their lives would make their lives smaller and maybe even less meaningful and fulfilling.

"Who would you say is your family now?" Erin S. Lavender-Stott and Katherine R. Allen posed that question in their in-depth interviews with thirteen lesbian and bisexual women, ages fifty-three through seventy-two, who had been single for at least five years.[327] The women were not legally married and not in a long-term romantic relationship. They had lived most of their adult lives before same-sex marriage was legalized in the US, and seven of them had been in heterosexual marriages before divorcing and forming same-sex relationships and then becoming single. Only one of the thirteen women disliked being single. The others described their single lives as happy, freeing, and psychologically rich.

In response to the question about family, they named conventional family members such as parents, siblings, ex-husbands, ex-partners, ex-in-laws, children, grandchildren, nieces, and nephews. But they also included other people they regarded as family, such as close friends (some of whom had been in their lives for decades) and children such as a neighbor's kids. Like so many queer people before them, their notions of family were expansive and inclusive. They had families they chose, not just conventional families.

Queer communities are among those who led the way in creating families of choice. Now, many others are following, including older single people, and not just those who are members of sexual or gender minorities. In later life, single people (divorced, widowed, or always single) are more likely than coupled people (married or cohabiting) to name a nonrelative as part of their family, a study of more than sixty-five hundred Dutch adults found.[328] Their unpartnered status does not limit the kinds of people they welcome into their lives, it expands it.

> ~~Friendships fill the gap for many who live alone.~~[329] —AARP report on solo agers
>
> **Fixed it!**
>
> *A spouse fills the gap for many who are married and don't have close friends.*

We Still Love Our Solitude

One characteristic that just about every person who is single at heart shares is a love of solitude. Age doesn't matter and neither does anything else. We love our solitude and we always have. We did not need to learn how to be alone. That comes naturally. Some of us had to learn to resist the insinuation that loving our alone time meant that there was something wrong with us. But by the time we get to our later years, we are long past that. We're not self-conscious anymore, if we ever were. We realize it is a great strength to flourish in solitude.

We have also benefited from building the kind of life that is especially likely to protect us from loneliness. As the studies I've already described have shown (and as other research has documented too), having a romantic partner in later life may not matter much at all, especially for women. What does matter is having supportive friends or family. Most people who are single at heart have been tending to their friends and relatives all along.

Even among people who are not single at heart, old age may be a time of lesser loneliness, and greater comfort with solitude, than fearmongering has led us to expect. Ask adults who are younger than sixty-five what they think their lives will be like when they are older, and about three in ten of them say that they worry that they will be lonely. But in the same study, fewer than two in ten who actually were sixty-five or older said that they were lonely.[330]

There is also evidence to suggest that, in the vast majority of instances, when older people are alone, that's what they want. In Vancouver, Canada, one hundred adults, ages fifty through eighty-five, were contacted several times a day for ten days, and asked each time whether they were alone or interacting with other people, and whether they wanted to be alone or with others. About 85 percent of the time, when they were alone, they wanted to be alone.[331]

Even during what could have been the worst of times for being old and alone, several months into the pandemic, the typical older adult did not seem to be suffering much from the imposed solitude. In the UK, more than two thousand people from three age groups (adolescents, middle-aged, and old) were asked to describe a recent experience when they were alone.[332] The people most likely to describe feeling at peace in their solitude were the oldest ones, sixty-five and older. They were less likely than the adolescents (ages thirteen to sixteen) to complain that they had nothing to do. Only 2 percent of the oldest participants said that they felt cut off from other people. More than half of both the oldest adults and the middle-aged adults (ages thirty-five to fifty-five) talked about the freedom they enjoyed when they were alone. They said that they liked their own company, and that they appreciated getting to do what they wanted, free of any social pressures. Fewer than a quarter of the adolescents said anything like that. In all three groups, the people who said they liked the freedom they had when they were alone were more at peace in their solitude than the people who said nothing about that. But the oldest people seemed to benefit the most. No one was more at peace in solitude than the oldest adults who said that when they were alone, they felt comfortable with themselves and free.

For decades, G. Clare Wenger and Vanessa Burholt of the University of Wales studied older people (sixty-five and older) in rural Wales, trying to understand the complex interplay between social isolation and loneliness. [333] To count as socially isolated, the participants had to meet more than one criterion—for example, they lived alone *and* they never went out of the house, or they had no close relatives and no phone. For some elders, the psychology of social isolation was just what anyone would expect—if they were isolated, they felt lonely, and if they weren't, they didn't. But the researchers also found seniors who had ample social connections and still felt lonely, and most intriguingly, they talked to people who, by objective measures, were isolated, but did not feel lonely. The most isolated among them had always kept to themselves, though others did have some interactions with friends or neighbors. Very few of them had children. On Christmas, some were alone—because that was their favorite way to celebrate. I don't know what the researchers expected when they showed up in person to interview these people, but what they reported afterward is that they often found them to be cheerful and pleasant. They were people who enjoyed their own company. One man who was profiled in the report said that he missed his wife who had died twenty-two years earlier. At eighty-four, though, he was still working as a gardener, and he was never lonely. I don't know if he would have identified as single at heart, but with regard to the way he has flourished in his solitude, he is surely one of us.

I'm not trying to dismiss the pain of people who truly are lonely. That's an important issue and needs to be taken seriously. But it would be misguided and counterproductive to assume that all, or even most, old people are lonely. Some savor their solitude, and among the single at heart, all of us do. We value having just the right mix of time alone and time with other people.

Our Homes Are Still Our Sanctuaries

When I renovated my house, I had quiet words with my builders and so now have a staircase which could easily be removed and replaced with a lift (elevator) and a bathroom which could be converted to a wet room with a sliding door. So hopefully I will be able to stay in this house, which I love, for most if not all of my life.
—Carla (thirty-three, Essex, England)

The AARP survey of solo agers found that they mostly felt good about living alone; 60 percent associated it with being independent.[334] So too do the single at heart, probably in even greater numbers. Compared to people who are not single at heart, more of us live alone, and we want to continue living alone, in our own homes, for as long as we possibly can.

Carla, quoted above, was decades away from old age, but she loves her solitude and loves her home, and at thirty-three, she was already thinking ahead to how she could arrange to stay there for as long as possible. Hers is another example of how we who are single at heart invest in our single lives throughout our lives, upping the odds that we will continue to live the life we want as we grow old.

Some who are single at heart prefer to live with others. Regardless, what we all want as we grow older is the freedom to continue to live as we choose. There is evidence that in China, in old age, single people are more likely than married people to live the way they want to live. In a study of more than fifteen thousand older adults in China, Melanie D. Sereny and Danan

Gu asked the elders which living arrangement they preferred (for example: alone, with a spouse, with children, in an institution), then compared their answers to how they were actually living.[335] They found that the elders who were not married were more likely than the married ones to be living the way they wanted to be. "Traditional Chinese older adults are expected to live in the community and to live with family members," Sereny and Gu explained. Yet, some preferred to live alone. The married seniors who were not living as they wished were often living with their children when they only wanted to be living with their spouse.

Our Role Models

A single person I look up to is my friend Sue, she's seventy-seven and we first met at work in 2007 and have been friends ever since. We talk on the phone a few times a month, mark each other's birthdays, etc. She's been single for a few decades, after two divorces earlier in her life decided she wouldn't want to live any other way than single after those experiences. She's very engaged with life, with multiple hobbies like bird-watching and gardening, and is passionate about politics and the environment. She is the antidote to the single scare story of " what will happen to you when you're old?" and that always inspires me, especially considering she has a chronic health condition that limits her mobility. To this day she still lives alone.

–Lucas Bradley (thirty-seven)

What If We Need Help?

"Who will care for you?" The question serves both to convey a real concern and also to criticize and goad. When addressed toward a younger woman, it aims to convince her to be sensible and marry, part of a broader process of gender socialization, sensitizing girls to feel that marriage will bring them patriarchal protection and security.[336]

–Sarah Lamb, *Being Single in India*

Old age is not what it used to be. Thanks to advances in medical science and in public health, in many nations, more people are staying healthy and active for more years than ever before (pandemics aside). When I was growing up, some of the sixty-five-year-olds looked more like today's eighty-year-olds. Perceptions haven't caught up. Adults in the US under the age of sixty-five, when asked what they expect to happen to them when they are older, anticipate a more dire old age than people who actually are sixty-five and older are experiencing. For example, in a Pew Research Center survey, 57 percent of the younger adults expected to experience memory loss, while only 25 percent of adults ages sixty and older actually were experiencing memory loss. Forty-two percent expected to have a serious illness; that was twice the number of older adults in the survey who did have a serious illness. Twenty-four percent expected to be a burden, more than twice as many as the 10 percent of older adults who thought they actually were a burden.[337]

One answer to the question of who will care for us, then, is that for a longer time than is typically anticipated, many of us may not need much help. But what happens when we do?

There is a specific woman that I have been emailing every morning for the past seven or eight years. It started off with just an email to let each other know that we are still alive and well as we both live alone. Over the years those emails have become a safe place for both of us. I was the first to know of her cancer diagnosis, and the only person for a period of time. While she had other friends that were retired and could stop by to help with things, it was me that she would pour her soul (depression and all) out to. She is much better now and has told me numerous times how much it helped knowing she had someone she could say anything to and knew it would never go anywhere. I know that if the time comes when I need someone she would be there for me, as would a few other friends.
—Kendra (sixty-nine, San Francisco, California)

In one of the most famous television ads of all time, an elderly woman, Mrs. Fletcher, is splayed on the floor of her bathroom, her upended walker beside her. "I've fallen and I can't get up," she cries. But she will be fine, because she has a medical alert device that she can use to call for help. The ad went viral. It has been referenced on popular television shows, and repeatedly spoofed.

It is no joke, though, when people try to use examples like that to try to frighten people who want to live alone. What if you fall and no one is there? What if you have a stroke? What if you suddenly become ill and can't reach your phone? What if, what if, what if, what if. Don't single people realize that they need to get married, or at least couple up and live with a partner for their own safety?

I have heard that argument presented to me in all seriousness. Sure, I love being single and living alone, but someday something is going to happen, I am told, and then I'm going to wish I were married.

It is an odd argument, that I should spend my entire adult life living in a way I don't want to live, married to someone when I want to be single, just so I will have a romantic partner to swoop in and save me when I've fallen and can't get up. (I think that's called using someone.) It's interesting that the person made famous in the ad was "Mrs." Fletcher. She wasn't saved by her spouse. Having a romantic partner, even a young and healthy one, is no guarantee that they will be there when you fall. Romantic partners often have jobs. Sometimes they travel. Sometimes they go out to do errands or get some exercise. And while it is true that a romantic partner who is away might still check in every day and would know if something seemed wrong, Kendra (quoted above) arranged for the same system of daily check-ins with a friend.

I think the ad is right. If you want to feel assured that you will be able to get help when you need it, forget a spouse. Your best bet may well be some kind of medical alert device. Joan, (seventy-three, Newark, Delaware) has one in place:

I have a Medical Guardian system that allows me to push a button and, if I don't answer when someone tries to call me, they call my contact people and send in first responders. I also have a key box on my door, like the ones realtors use, and the alarm company would give the code to first responders so they can get in. Several friends also have that code. As that suggests, I've certainly contemplated the implications of aging alone, and have taken reasonable precautions.

Scaremongering about growing old without a spouse rarely focuses only on one-time experiences, such as taking a fall. The what-ifs are much more sweeping: What will happen to me, a person with no committed romantic partner (and no children either), when I become seriously ill or injured and need a lot of help for a long time?

Kristin (fifty-five, Bellingham, Washington), an avid cyclist, was in her happy place. She was riding her beloved bicycle, Silver, along the side of the road on her way to get takeout from her favorite Thai restaurant. In an instant, a distracted driver barreled into her, sending her careening down a hill. By the time she reached the bottom, her upper arm bone was shattered, her shoulder bone fractured, and every rib on one side of her body broken. She had two spinal fractures, a fractured skull, a torn liver, collapsed lungs, and a collapsed carotid artery. One of her hands dangled from her arm. The crash scene was so horrifying, officials assumed she had died.

Kristin was forty-six at the time, and living alone. She didn't have a romantic partner. She had been married, but the relationship had ended years ago. She had family, but not nearby. She had no kids. Some would say she had no one at all. Who would be there for her now?

Kristin's story is one that unnerves many who might otherwise be drawn to single life. Single people often worry about lesser challenges, such as finding someone to stay with them during an outpatient medical procedure. Kristin was looking at six weeks of hospitalization, followed by three months of in-home care, then six months of outpatient rehab. In medical journals, doctors have speculated, without evidence, that single people facing daunting diagnoses and treatment regimens may lack the "fighting spirit" they need to survive.[338] They don't know Kristin.

Kristin's parents flew in to be at her side, worried not just about her catastrophic injuries, but the possibility that she would be all alone. But Kristin was a devoted volunteer at the local animal shelter, and her fellow volunteers showed up in droves. She had made friends in a trivia league; they came too. So did other friends and several of her neighbors. Even her ex was there for her. So many people wanted to visit Kristin that the hospital staff had to reschedule them or shoo them away. Today she is back to bicycling, volunteering, writing, and pursuing her work as an artisan, with even more devoted friends than before.

Did Kristin survive despite the fact that she was single? I think she thrived *because* she was single—not just single but single at heart. She had been married before, but she found that life isolating and depressing. Later, without a romantic partner at the center of her life expecting to be prioritized and compromised for, Kristin was free to invest as much time and emotional energy into as many different people as she wanted. She didn't have to be sexually or romantically involved with another person to treat them with great care and attentiveness, and to have that care and attentiveness returned when she needed it. Fellow volunteers, game-night buddies, friends, neighbors, and even animals were all welcomed into Kristin's warm embrace. She didn't have The One, she had The Ones, and that was her secret strength.

Does Kristin's story strike you as extraordinary? Kristin is, for sure, an extraordinary person. But the story of single people getting the help that they need may only seem uncommon because it is so rarely told.

Kristin's story was not the only one I could have chosen to show how the single at heart are cared for when they need a lot of help over a long period of time. Joan (seventy-three, Newark, Delaware) was diagnosed with Stage 4 cancer when she was sixty-five. She had no spouse or romantic partner and no kids, and her parents had died. However, she had a lifetime of cherished friends, and some cousins too. They were there for her every step of the way. In my research for *How We Live Now*, I interviewed Lucy, who was seventy-one when she was diagnosed with cancer. Like Joan, she had never been married and had no children and her parents were deceased. Her remaining relatives lived eight hundred miles away. She did have people who were there for her, though—"Lucy's Angels," a staggering forty-nine friends who wanted to help.

Friends are not obligated to show up for each other in the way that a spouse or committed romantic partner is. That is one of the reasons why people who have such a partner can feel more secure that they will be cared for than single people do. Their security is fragile, though, and not just because romantic partners are not always available to help or able to do so. Sometimes, when one person in a married couple faces serious health problems, the other one flees.

A study of 2,701 American marriages showed that when a wife (but not a husband) became seriously ill, the likelihood of divorce increased.[339] In a study of nearly eight thousand American married couples, the chances of divorce increased if a husband (but not a wife) became limited in the kinds of work he could do because of his health.[340]

Even when a spouse does stand by a partner who becomes seriously ill, they are not always all that helpful. A study of 102 women with breast cancer found that their significant others (most of whom were husbands) were helpful when the women had trouble with physical tasks, such as lifting, carrying, or reaching things. However, when the women became more emotionally distressed, their significant others became less supportive. When they did try to help, their attempts were ineffective—the women did not feel any less distressed and they did not recover any more quickly.[341]

A study of more than thirty-eight hundred American women with breast cancer showed that having a spouse did nothing for the women's likelihood of surviving.[342] It was the women who had close friends, relatives, or children who were most likely to still be alive up to twelve years after their diagnosis. The married women had The One and that did not save them. The women who had The Ones (friends, relatives, or children) did better.

Of course, not all married or coupled people practice intensive coupling, looking to their partner to be the one and only important person in their life, the person to fulfill all their wishes and needs. Those who do so, though, are most likely to be at risk. In a British study, for example, they were less likely to have good mental health than the coupled people who had other confidants and companions.[343]

The advantages of having The Ones rather than The One are not just psychological. In practical ways too, multilayered support systems can provide protection. If someone in Kristin's network had other commitments or fell ill or was simply in a bad place emotionally, Kristin was not as vulnerable as she might have been if she had been counting only on a spouse for all of her support needs. The people providing the support benefit too, emotionally and practically, when the sole or primary burden is not on them. They can provide the kind of help they want to give, when they are able to provide it, without worrying that if they don't step up, no one else will. When Lucy's forty-nine angels volunteered to help, they had to figure out on their own a system for coordinating. Now there are online platforms that facilitate that, such as CaringBridge.org and LotsaHelpingHands.com.

In addition to the Magical Mythical Romantic Partner, one other kind of person is also heralded as a key to a secure old age, a way of assuring ourselves that there will be someone there to care for us when we need help: grown children. They are the Savior Children. Some people who are single at heart have children, but more of us do not.

Like romantic partners, grown children also have lives. They are not always available to help or able to help. Some live nowhere near their parents. Others would not help even if they did live nearby. In the US, for example, it is estimated that more than one-quarter of adults are estranged from a family member.[344]

In a survey conducted in three nations, grown children were asked how much help their parents actually needed.[345] In Italy, only 18 percent whose parents were between ages sixty-five and seventy-four said that their parents needed help handling their affairs or caring for themselves. In the US, 15 percent said the same, and in Germany, only 11 percent did. Of the parents who were even older than that (seventy-five and older), more of them needed help, but again, most did not. In Italy, 48 percent of grown children said that their parents who were seventy-five or older needed help handling their affairs or caring for themselves. In the US and Germany, the percentages were just 33 and 29, respectively.

As for financial assistance, in all three countries, aging parents are much more likely to be helping their adult children than vice versa. In the US and Germany, twice as many parents are helping their children financially than receiving help from them, and in Italy, three times as many are giving money to their grown children than receiving it.

Some older parents feel better if they live with or near their grown children, perhaps in part because they feel reassured that those kids will be available to help if needed. In a study of widowed adults in the US who were sixty-five and older, those who lived with their offspring or near them felt less distressed than those whose offspring lived more than an hour's drive away, if they had a good relationship.[346] But there were costs too. The widowed parents who lived with their adult children were less likely to see friends, relatives, or neighbors. They missed out on those other possible sources of companionship and support.

In some countries, filial devotion is expected. In India, for example, adult children are required by law to pay their parents a monthly allowance. It is commonplace there for aging parents to live with their grown children and their families. But among economically secure widows living in urban areas of India, sociologist Jagriti Gangopadhyay is finding, some are opting to live alone instead.[347] They appreciate the greater freedom and control over their lives that comes with having a place of their own. They are still in close touch with their kids, and often report that their relationships with them are stronger and less emotionally fraught because they are not living with them. When they need help, they rely on drivers, maids, and other hired help.

People in India who have no children do not get the monthly allowances from grown children that Indian parents can count on, and they don't have the possibility of getting emotional support from offspring either. What if they also have no spouse or romantic partner, and they are living alone in the midst of a pandemic? During the COVID-19 lockdown, women's studies scholar Ketaki Chowkhani interviewed people between the ages of forty and fifty who were not married and not in a romantic relationship, had no children, and were living alone.[348] Unlike the widows Gangopadhyay studied, these long-term single people were relying mostly on networks of friends, relatives, chosen family members, and work colleagues, rather than paid help. Even when they could not see those people in person, they stayed connected in other ways. They were also skilled at flourishing in their solitude. They cared for themselves and maintained their health and well-being by eating right, exercising, getting enough sleep, having a routine, enjoying their favorite forms of entertainment, and pursuing their creative and spiritual interests.

If and when there comes a time when we are no longer able to care for ourselves on our own, the single at heart may need to relinquish some of our cherished solitude and independence. Those of us who love living alone may need to make room for another person in our home. We won't have a spouse and many of us will not have children, but that doesn't necessarily mean that we will have no one. As I touched on earlier, some single people are already making plans to share a home with friends when they get older, and others have moved in together even before they have grown old. We don't have to figure it out on our own if we don't want to. New and innovative arrangements are being created all the time, such as those that pair older people who have homes and need help with younger people who need a place to stay and want to help.

Alternatively, we may need to, or prefer to, move into accommodations such as assisted living or other special facilities such as memory care if we are dealing with dementia. Somewhere along the way we may also need an advocate who will look out for us when we are hospitalized and even when we are not. What we may need most if we are no longer able to care for ourselves are financial resources. With enough money, we can hire an advocate, move into assisted living, or employ home health aides or live-in help. Those costs can be daunting, though, and as I'll show in the next chapter, single people are often systematically—and unfairly—disadvantaged financially throughout our lives. Until needed reforms are in place, we may have to be more attentive to money matters, and from an earlier age, than our more privileged peers.

~~Who will be there for you?~~

Fixed it!

Who will be there for you if you make your spouse or romantic partner the center of your universe, demote everyone else, and then that person is gone?

Dying Alone? We're Not Afraid of That

There used to be a fashion for scaremongering surveys about single women, saying things like: "Eight out of ten women are going to die alone, surrounded by seventeen cats." But to that I would mentally add: "Or it could all go horribly wrong."[349]
—Barbara Ellen, "Loneliness is one thing, a happy loner quite another"

The single at heart just aren't afraid of being alone. We are not afraid of spending a lot of time alone, going to sleep alone, waking up alone, dining alone, traveling alone, living alone, or aging alone. And we are not afraid of dying alone. When I asked the single at heart people who shared their life stories with me if they were afraid of dying alone, several gave some version of what Eleanore (sixty-four, Sydney, Australia) said: "I've never understood the dying alone thing."

It made no sense to worry about it, some explained, because everyone dies alone. Carla (thirty-three, Essex, England) put it this way: "Ultimately, you can be in a roomful of people who love you and you still have to take that final step over on your own." Julie (forty-four, Raleigh, North Carolina) said she wouldn't be alone: "I have Jesus, always."

"Even if you spend your entire life married, only one person in a couple is going to have their spouse at their side at the time of death," Sonya (forty-seven, Parkersburg, West Virginia) said, echoing a point others made as well. In a way, Sonya's perspective is optimistic. Spending your entire life married is no guarantee that either spouse will have the other at their side when they die—or anyone else. My father died on the bathroom floor of a hospital room when an aneurysm burst. I don't know how long he lay there alone before a nurse found him and a doctor tried to revive him. He had lived his life in the way that is respected and celebrated and is supposed to protect against dying alone: he was married to my mom for his entire adult life, and he had four grown kids who would have done anything for him—and grandkids too. But it was after midnight when he died, and my mother had left his room and gone home an hour or so earlier. None of the kids or grandkids were in town.

A whole industry of death doulas, hospice volunteers, and other specialists has now cropped up to ensure that No One Dies Alone (NODA). But scholars and journalists who study death and dying have found that some people want to die alone. It is their choice, their own version of a good death. In researching her book, *Dying Alone: Challenging Assumptions*, the sociologist Glenys Caswell talked to older people in the UK who lived alone about their wishes.[350] She also interviewed bereaved people about their experiences, as well as palliative care nurses, hospice workers, funeral directors, and coroners. The older people living alone said that they valued their independence, and they were more concerned about threats to that independence (such as needing care) than about dying alone. In her study of the kinds of deaths that get so much media attention and public pity, people whose bodies are found days or even years after they died, Caswell reported, "In most cases, the death was of a private person who liked their own company."

Both Caswell and Ann Neumann, author of *The Good Death*, pointed to a phenomenon that just about every hospice worker and palliative nurse has witnessed: the dying patient has loved ones sitting vigil; then, just when they step outside the room for a moment, the patient dies.[351] A single mother who wrote a guest post for one of my blogs under the name "Think Again" shared, "I hope that my children are at my bedside, and they have a chance to say goodbye, but I don't want either of them to feel the pressure of holding my hand 24/7 until my time comes."[352] She also wrote that she will not need their presence, or anyone else's, to know that she is loved. "No matter where I am, if I'm alone or surrounded by strangers, it doesn't change what's in my heart, and what's in the hearts of those I love."

Because the single at heart have typically tended to The Ones their whole life, they are unlikely to die alone if they don't want to. But some do want to, or would be at peace with it if it happened that way. David (sixty-five, Austin, Texas) said, "I would actually rather face death knowingly and with interest and not be distracted by reacting to or comforting others who are in an emotional state concerning my passing." Joan (seventy-three, Newark, Delaware) expressed similar sentiments: "My focus is on not dying when I might have survived if the necessary help had come soon enough, but once I am actively dying, I don't want anyone chattering in my ear. I'd be perfectly happy to have it happen when I'm alone." Marie (forty-six, Northern California) said, "If I died alone tomorrow, I would transcend this plane in the presence of self-love." And finally, Donna (forty-nine, Seattle, Washington) said, "I'm like an old country dog. When it's my time, I want to crawl under the deck and be alone when it happens."

Our Role Models

I first met Dave and Rex back in the '80s when we all lived on the same floor of our college dorm. The three of us bonded over late-night runs to the all-night doughnut shop near campus and frequent movie screenings of *Revenge of the Nerds* and *Monty Python's The Meaning of Life.*

Thirty-five years later, Dave was lying in a hospital bed on life support after having contracted meningitis. I called Rex who was at his bedside. The medical science, he told me, indicated Dave had already left us. The machines were scheduled to be turned off the following day once his parents arrived. Rex put the phone on speaker so I could say goodbye.

Rex did this for all of Dave's friends who phoned him.

The three of us never married or had children. But soon after graduating from college, Dave had gotten involved in the Big Brother program. Years later, he became a mentor in DeMolay International, an organization for boys aged twelve to twenty-one. Some of the people calling Rex at the hospital were people Dave had mentored as teenagers. And as Rex put the phone on speaker, he heard caller after caller describe how much Dave had meant to them, including how he had helped shape these young adults from their teen years into the grown men they had become. He was, in his own way, a role model.

Married or single, with or without children of our own, we can all have an impact and leave a legacy.

—Elliott Lewis (Syracuse, New York)

For most single people, dying alone will never be an issue. As I've discussed previously, single people typically have robust networks of friends and relatives who are emotionally meaningful to them. If they are not just single but also single at heart, they have not sidelined the important people in their lives in order to prioritize a romantic partner. Those people will likely be there for them at the end if they want them to be. And, as Elliott's story illustrates, sometimes single people who do not have children of their own have been mentors and role models to other young people, whose grateful and loving voices may be among the last they hear.

Old and Married: Some Want What the Single at Heart Have

I lived alone but I was less lonely than I had been earlier in my life. People made judgments; I didn't heed them. Some asked questions; I didn't answer them. Others—mainly women—understood, because they, too, had experienced the unbearable loneliness of marriage.[353]
—Ruth Wilson, *The Jane Austen Remedy*

Ruth Wilson had been married fifty years when she moved to a cottage to live on her own. "I longed to make decisions without being challenged, to be the one who sometimes had the last word," she explained. "I was especially tired of being surrounded by people whose values I could no longer pretend to share."[354] She stayed married, but she embraced what the single at heart find so dear—solitude, space, the freedom to be the decider, to live by her own values, and to welcome into her life the kinds of people she wanted in her life and not the ones she didn't. She described that time as "the best years of my life."[355]

Since reaching a peak in 1980, the divorce rate in the US has declined. There's an important exception, though—among those fifty and older, the rates doubled between 1990 and 2015.[356] Young people (under forty) still divorce at higher rates overall, but their likelihood of divorcing is decreasing while older people's is increasing. Something else is striking about the fifty-and-older crowd: very substantial numbers of them are staying single. Susan L. Brown and her colleagues followed Americans in that age group for ten years after they divorced and found that 62 percent of the men and 77 percent of the women had not remarried and they had not cohabited either.[357] Some of them may have wanted to become coupled again but just never found the right person. For others, after years of following the conventional life path, stepping off it to savor the best of single life may have felt like a glorious reward.

Generally, divorce rates are higher among people who have been married for a shorter time. Nonetheless, in 2015, of the people fifty and older who had divorced, one-third of them had been married for at least thirty years.[358] Deirdre Bair wanted to understand why people divorced late in life after decades of marriage, so she interviewed 310 people who had done so. Here's Bair's description of what they told her: "Most of them mentioned 'freedom.' Another word I heard a lot was 'control': people wanted it for themselves for the rest of their lives. . . . Women and men alike wanted time to find out who they were."[359]

Like people who are single at heart, these people who ended long-lasting marriages wanted their freedom, they wanted to be the deciders, and they wanted to live authentically. "To them," Bair said, "divorce meant not failure and shame, but opportunity."[360]

No Regrets

I wish I'd had the courage to live a life true to myself,
not the life others expected of me.[361]
—The number one regret of the dying, as reported by
Bronnie Ware in *The Top Five Regrets of the Dying*

Like anyone else, we who are single at heart may have all sorts of regrets as we lay dying, but we will be spared the most common and the most fundamental regret of all—living the life we were supposed to live, instead of our most authentic life. We defied one of the most powerful norms about how to live— we never did look for The One and then organize the rest of our lives around that person. Instead we were true to ourselves. We lovingly embraced our single lives. We invested in ourselves. We invested in The Ones. At the end, with regard to the matter of authenticity, we will be at peace.

When the single at heart shared with me their expectations about how they will look back at their lives, they expressed confidence and pride, not regret. Claudia (sixty-nine, Washington, DC), for example, said, "I believe that when I am gasping my last few breaths, as I review all the things I've done, places I've been, that I will feel that I had a life, and that I lived it." Claudia has not put off the pursuit of her dreams in hopes of finding a romantic partner to pursue them with her. Like other people who are single at heart, she is living her psychologically rich life fully, joyfully, and authentically.

I can also tell you about an actual deathbed experience of one of my beloved single at heart study participants. Carol, the person I described who became a "rock chick" in London at fifty-one, beat cancer multiple times over the course of her adult life. When it recurred again before she turned sixty, she once again tried every treatment available, but that time, it was to no avail. Her doctors told her there was nothing more they could do. She called to tell me the terrible news. We talked and we cried and we told each other how much we meant to each other. When I hung up, I felt devastated. But I also felt so tremendously proud of Carol. She lived a good life, she knew she lived a good life, and she was at peace.

In one of the last emails she sent to me, as she lay dying, Carol told me that she was asked if she wanted to talk to a psychologist. She said that she didn't think she needed to, but did so anyway. Afterward, the psychologist agreed with Carol—she did not need a therapist. "She said that I was a fully self-actualized person," Carol told me. "I was thrilled. That was my goal in life and I have achieved it."

Advice For the Single at Heart

To continue living your full and fulfilling life into old age, maintain your ties with people you enjoy having in your life. Your attention to "The Ones" instead of just "The One" can be a special strength throughout your life, but perhaps even more so as you age. You aren't going to end up on your own for the first time, wondering how you will ever manage. You've been managing—and thriving—for decades.

Take care of yourself in whatever ways work best for you. Self-care is not just an indulgence; it is an investment in your health and happiness and peace of mind.

Think ahead to the kinds of living arrangements that will be most suitable as you age. If you want to continue to live in a place of your own as long as possible, look for a place that is age-friendly or modify your own place. Do you prefer to live with others or near them in an intentional community? Look into shared housing or cohousing communities. Do you have friends who have fantasized about living together once you are older? Do you share those fantasies? If so, see if your friends are serious and start planning.

Think about location too. Do you want to live close to shops, services, and public transportation? Do you want to live in a certain climate? Do you want to live somewhere with particularly good services for older people? Do you need to be near medical facilities?

Tend to your financial needs. Pay off your debts if you can. If, in later life, you need long-term care or if you want to move to a place such as assisted living, that can be very expensive in many places. Look for expert advice on matters such as long-term care insurance and financial planning.

Prepare your will and other documents such as a power of attorney and an advance care directive. Be sure that the relevant people have what they will need if they have to take over for you, such as the names of your doctors, your bank records and passwords, and a list of the bills that need to be paid.

Think about your legacy. Without a spouse who expects to be your beneficiary, you have the opportunity to continue to honor the people and causes you care about even after you are gone.

Feel proud of yourself for your enduring love of solitude. That fear of spending time alone that worries so many other people as they look toward their later years is something that will never plague you.

Continue to make the most of your freedom to live your most joyful, psychologically rich, and authentic single life. If you want to follow in the footsteps of people like Barbara Hillary, who were still planning their next adventures as they approached their nineties, don't let anyone dissuade you! You've got this.

For Our Allies

As your single at heart friends and family enter their older years, tune into what they love to do and acknowledge and support those interests. If they need help with transportation or other practical tasks, offer to provide it; if you need help, ask them.

If you are an educator, lead the way in teaching your students about the single people who are flourishing in later life, especially those who have been single their whole lives. If you are a member of the creative class, feature older single people who are thriving (and not looking to unsingle themselves!) in your novels, short stories, screenplays, poems, song lyrics, and other artwork. Think about what they have learned about life from their special vantage point outside of the conventional ways of living. That's also a good perspective for mental health professionals, who are in a special position to validate the wisdom of people who have been single for decades and who have had the strength to triumph over all the singlism they have endured.

If you are a builder, an architect, a city planner, or a policymaker, think about how to design buildings, residences, public spaces, and communities that are welcoming to the growing numbers of people who are single in their later years. Some want to live alone in a home and in a neighborhood that is easy to navigate as they grow older. Others want to live with other people, in places where each adult has their own ample space, and no one is relegated to a room designed for a child.

If you are a health care professional recommending a surgery, outpatient procedure, or other treatment, ask about our resources and our needs rather than just making assumptions. Some single people will need transportation or someone to stay with them if that is a requirement. Others will have friends or relatives who are happy to help, and those people will need to be acknowledged and accepted in those roles by nurses and other personnel just as spouses and grown children are. Remember too that these kinds of concerns are not specific to single people or people without grown children. Coupled people and parents may have partners and children who are unable to help (perhaps because of their own health issues) or unavailable to help (as, for example, when grown children have other commitments or live far away) or unwilling to help.

To all of our allies, don't refer to all older women as "grandmothers." Many are not mothers or grandmothers, and even among those who are, not all want to be defined by that role.

For People Who Are Intrigued by Single Life, But Have Concerns

The best way to decide about embracing single life if you are unsure about it is to try it out. Act like you really are single at heart. That means *investing in yourself* (pursuing what matters to you, taking good care of yourself, developing your skills and planning for a life of your own rather than counting on someone else) and *investing in others* (valuing the people you care about and not just the people, such as a romantic partner, that you are told you should care about). That can only redound to your benefit, even if you ultimately decide that a more conventional coupled life is what you want.

If single life sounds great to you, don't let anyone dissuade you with their dire predictions of what will potentially befall you in old age. Untold numbers of people who embraced their single lives have already proved them wrong. Think instead of what you will miss if you believe that single life is your best life, but you never choose to live that life.

9

The Resistance

In May 2021, an email from "Youk Unt Unupalam" appeared in my inbox:

> Hi Bella,
>
> Just want to let you know that single people are inferior in every way. They're worthless, useless, lazy and stupid. There's nothing I hate like single people. Anyone single is completely defective, otherwise someone would love them.
>
> Now, Bella, I know you found some micro/macro aggressions there, but I want you to use all of your Harvard skills to understand it's entirely your fault. You're single, therefore you suck.
>
> You suck because you're single. Say it out loud. You are nothing. Worthless.

Yes, I know, he's a troll. Don't feed the trolls. I didn't respond, but I am interested in why someone like "Youk" would compose such a vile message and send it to someone he doesn't even know. I don't think he despises me, and wants me to know that he despises me, because I am single. He wants to devastate me because I am *happily* single, and want to stay that way. Also, I won't shut up about it.

My troll is upset by some of the very qualities that make me who I am. At the heart of being single at heart is the experience of single life as a joyful place, a place where we want to stay because, for us, no other way of living could ever be so meaningful, fulfilling, or psychologically rich. By living single, we get to honor who we really are. Free from trying to organize our lives around a romantic partner the way we know we are supposed to, the way that would sap our spirit and make our lives feel fake, we instead get to flourish.

Decades ago, when I first started studying attitudes toward single people, I knew that single people were at risk for being stereotyped and stigmatized, and my own research confirmed that.[362] And yet, deep down, I think I expected to be protected from a lot of that negativity by my own happiness. I have never once harangued my friends with "poor me" stories of single life or pleaded with them to find someone—anyone!—for me. I have never called my mother on some milestone birthday and cried about "still" being single.

I'm the happy single person! Shouldn't that be a good thing? One of the most surprising discoveries in all my years of living single and studying single people is that it is not.

My own expressions of happiness, I have learned, are sometimes viewed as suspect. If I were coupled, I could say that I was happy and no one would second-guess me; in fact, they'd probably already assume as much before I even said a word.

Emotional Resistance: Refusing to Believe We Really Are Happy

As a single person, I'm not supposed to be happy. I've been hearing that my whole life, and not just from the relentless cultural messaging in which "you deserve to be happy" means that you should commit to a romantic partner, and "happily ever after" means you already did. My colleagues and I, in one study after another, have found the same presumption that single people just aren't happy, not like those married or coupled people.[363] Sometimes we ask people to tell us the characteristics that come to mind when they think about single people or married people. Happiness is something that comes to mind more often when the participants in our research are asked to list the characteristics of married people than when they are asked to describe single people.

In other studies, we created pairs of brief biographical sketches of people that were identical in every way, except that in one, the person was said to be single, and in the other, married. We showed each of our participants one of the two versions and asked them to tell us how happy they thought the person was, and how happy the person would say they were. They consistently rated the married person as happier than the single person, even though both had identical biographies except for their marital status.

It was actually worse than that. They thought that the single people, more so than the married ones, would say that they were happier than they really were. They were discounting single people's claims to their own happiness.

I know the feeling. I've been on a lot of podcasts. On one of them, after an hour of prerecording a lively and engaging conversation, the podcast host said, "You are the happiest person I have ever interviewed." I was beaming! Then she paused for a moment and added, "or at least you present that way."

When my colleagues and I first started finding that people view single people as less happy than married people, and think that if only they would marry, they would become lastingly happier, we thought they might be assuming that single people don't have anyone in their lives. We did another study in which we created new profiles of single (and married) people, making it clear that they had a circle of longtime friends, were close to their siblings, and were friendly with their neighbors. It didn't matter. Our participants still overwhelmingly thought the single people weren't as happy as the married people, and that when single people said they were happy, they were exaggerating.

We tried again. Maybe they thought single people were selfish, so we did another version of the study that specified that the people they were judging were remarkably altruistic. That didn't matter either. It also didn't help to describe the people in the profiles as having great career accomplishments or impressive material success. No, no, no, no, no, our participants insisted: single people aren't really all that happy; married people are. Single people might say they are happy, but you can't really believe them.[364]

It is as if they thought that getting married magically transforms a miserable single person into a blissfully happy coupled person. Only it doesn't. More than a dozen studies have followed the same people over years of their lives to see if they become lastingly happier after they marry than they were before. They don't.[365] Sometimes they experience a brief increase in happiness around the time of the wedding, but over time they go back to the same level of happiness they experienced when they were single. And that brief uptick in happiness early on, sometimes called "the honeymoon effect," is experienced primarily by those people who married and stayed married. The couples who were headed toward divorce were, on average, already becoming less happy as their wedding day approached, rather than happier.

In those studies, the participants were already happy when they were single. On average, their happiness ratings were clearly on the happy end of the rating scales. That's been true in countless other studies too, in which single people were asked about their happiness at just one point in time. Probably more than a million single people have participated in studies like that. I have yet to find even one study in which single people, on average, are unhappy. Of course, there are some single people who are unhappy (just as there are some coupled people who are unhappy), but they are the exceptions. If there is one bottom line about the happiness of single people, it is this: single people are happy. And I'm not just talking about people who are single at heart. Averaging across all single people, happiness rules.

Social scientists have had a hand in promoting the narrative that getting married makes people happy. They often claim that married people are happier than single people, without acknowledging what is wrong with that claim.[366] For example, single and married people differ in many ways other than their marital status, and maybe those differences, rather than marital status, account for the differences in happiness. Also, when researchers compare people who are currently married to those who have always been single, they are ignoring all the people who got married and then got divorced; marriage had not made them happy. Perhaps most importantly, if marriage really did make people happier, then single people who marry should become reliably happier. But that's not what happens.

Our Happiness, and Our Commitment to Staying Single, Can Seem Threatening

An innocent explanation of the belief that single people aren't happy is that people just don't know any better. If they knew the truth about the actual happiness of single people, they might readily accept it. But they don't. As my studies (and my own experiences) showed, people don't accept single people's reports of their own happiness at face value. They insist that single people are saying they are happy when they really aren't. They seem *invested* in believing that single people cannot be happy, that they cannot really *want* to be single. If that's what's going on, then people will not just disbelieve single people who say they want to be single, they will also disparage them.

In two studies, one from the US[367] and the other from Israel,[368] that's exactly what happened. In brief biographical sketches, single people were described as either wanting to stay single or wanting to be coupled. The single people who wanted to stay single were not complaining about their life; they were not yearning to unsingle themselves. And yet it was those single people, rather than the single people who were pining for a partner, who were judged to be *less* happy and *less* secure. They were derogated in other ways too. They were deemed less warm, less sociable, and more self-centered. Most startlingly, the participants in the research expressed anger at the single people who had chosen to be single.

What is their offense? Single people who want to be single and who are happily single are challenging a cherished worldview that suffuses every corner of our lives, from fairy tales and popular culture to botched reports of the results of the latest study. It is a worldview and mythology that offers a nearly irresistible promise: *Get married and all the pieces of your life will fall in place; you will be happier and healthier than those single people; you will be morally superior too.* Many people want that myth to be true, and anyone who defies it will be resisted mightily.

Single people who don't want to be single can be just as devoted to the worldview of marital superiority as anyone else. Some are powerfully drawn to the prospect of finding their own "sex and everything else partner," my name for the person they can look to "for companionship, intimacy, caring, friendship, advice, the sharing of the tasks and finances of household and family, and just about everything else."[369] Find that one person and you're done. And now you're superior too. It's like magic.

Conventional coupling can feel democratic and fair, something that anyone can attain regardless of their background or position in life. But this is false; opportunities to find a suitable partner are not equally available to all.[370] For example, people with caregiving responsibilities, health problems, or onerous work schedules may not have much time or energy for dating. People who live in rural areas may have fewer potentially available local partners than people who live in cities. Systematic biases can also constrain opportunities. For instance, discriminatory criminalization, in which black men are more often incarcerated than white men when their offenses are comparable or even less severe, can result in fewer available partners for black women interested in black men. And yet, the perception that just about anyone can become coupled adds to the power and the appeal of the mythology of marriage and romantic coupling. Some (not all) people who are coupled are even more deeply invested than the reluctantly single in the myth of the superiority of people who are coupled. They did what they were supposed to do—they found that one special person and put that romantic partner at the center of their lives. They are accustomed to being admired and celebrated. They expect single people to look longingly not just at their partner, but their entire life. They feel entitled to our envy. Hearing instead that we are perfectly happy with our own single lives can enrage them.

University of Denver law professor Nancy Leong suggests another way in which people who choose to be single and want to stay single may be threatening to people who are coupled. The mere existence of those single people can compel coupled people "to contemplate what life might be like . . . without a partner . . . Perhaps it forces [them] to admit they are a little bit curious, or a little bit jealous. Or it might force them to convince themselves that they are not curious, or not jealous. The intensity of the attraction manifests itself in overt revulsion."[371]

I think she is right, but I am also reassured by other research showing that it is mostly only the insecurely coupled people who are inclined to feel jealous of the contently single and then react by denigrating them. The people who are secure in their own romantic relationship status and skills are less likely to disparage happy single people.[372] They may have no interest whatsoever in living single, but they do not feel threatened by people who do. They are our allies.

At this point in my life, I don't think anyone could ever make me feel bad about being single. I know that staying single is not, and never has been, a failure. It is how I live my most meaningful and fulfilling life. In fact, to me, defying all the pressures to lead a conventional coupled life, and not even pretending to want that life, is a victory and a source of pride.

I can, though, easily become infuriated on behalf of all the single people who have felt shamed for being single and who have been led to believe that the Magical Mythical Marital Partner is real. I have heard from psychotherapists whose single clients sometimes believe that they are unhappy because they are single, and if only they would marry, they really and truly would live happily ever after. I have heard from people who are single at heart who were unhappy when they tried to live a coupled life but kept trying because the cultural messaging about the supposedly transformative power of coupling is so relentless. That messaging is harmful. I'm especially exasperated when it is perpetrated by people who should know better, such as the social scientists who write deficit narratives of single life and do not acknowledge the scientifically documented ways in which many single people are flourishing. It would be easier on me emotionally if I didn't care; I hope I never get to that point.[373]

Marriage Has Become a Status Symbol and an Engine of Inequality

> Marriage for many . . . becomes a celebration of their
> personal achievements, a symbol of their success that they
> can celebrate with family and friends.[374]
> —Sociology professor Andrew Cherlin, "Degrees of Change: An
> Assessment of the Deinstitutionalization of Marriage Thesis"

In the 1950s in the US, just about everyone got married and stayed married. And they got married at the youngest ages ever recorded in Census Bureau records dating back to 1890: a low of 20.1 for women and 22.5 for men (as compared to 28.6 for women and 30.4 for men in 2021).[375] Marriage wasn't special, it was ordinary. It was just what people did.

Now, several decades into the twenty-first century, marriage has become the province of the people who are the most advantaged. In a 2014 survey, single women said that having a steady job was an important criterion for choosing a spouse or partner,[376] and in other research, cohabiting couples expressed a reluctance to marry if they did not feel that they were on firm financial footing.[377] As good jobs became less available and more precarious, financial security slipped beyond the reach of many who wanted to marry, and therefore marriage did too. As of 2015, 65 percent of US college graduates were married, compared to just 50 percent of those with high school degrees or less. Among people racialized as white, 54 percent were married, compared to just 30 percent racialized as black.[378]

In many instances, wedding celebrations have morphed from simple ceremonies with modest receptions to extravaganzas, sometimes extending over several days in far-flung destinations. They are, in essence, events for the affluent.

The people who are already privileged are most likely to marry, then those who do marry are showered with a whole panoply of additional advantages, way beyond all the wedding gifts they collect. At the federal level, there are hundreds of benefits and protections in the US reserved for those who are legally married.[379] At state and local levels too, laws often favor people who are married, and so do the policies and practices of workplaces, the marketplace, colleges and universities, and of course, religious institutions.[380]

In *Moving Past Marriage*, Jaclyn Geller, a literature professor who is not married and never has been, explored just some of the many rewards available only to people who are married.[381] Social Security is a big one. Professor Geller and her colleagues all pay into the Social Security system. When her married colleagues die, their spouses can receive their Social Security benefits. Eligible recipients include spouses who have never paid anything into the system, as well as every ex-spouse whose marriage to the deceased lasted at least ten years. Professor Geller's benefits, though, would go back into the system. She and all the other lifelong single people are subsidizing the benefits that go to the spouses and ex-spouses of married people.

The surviving spouses of her deceased colleagues would also receive a few hundred dollars toward final expenses. Because Professor Geller does not have a spouse or children, no one in her life, no matter how important she had been to them, will be eligible to receive that benefit. No paid funeral expenses for lifelong single people!

Inheritance is straightforward for the surviving spouse of a married person, even if the deceased dies without a will. The widowed person gets all the assets. Professor Geller could name beneficiaries in her will, but they would not get the tax breaks on inheritance taxes or estate taxes that those widows and widowers would receive.

Married people can open a spousal Individual Retirement Account; their spouse can tap into it early without incurring a penalty. Not so for lifelong single people, or anyone they name as a beneficiary; they pay early withdrawal fees. Spouses can also give each other huge monetary gifts without paying taxes. Single people have no such tax protections for comparable gifts to the people who mean the most to them.

Immigration rights, hospital visitation rights, and the privilege of not testifying against your spouse in criminal cases are just a few of the other federal benefits and protections that married people enjoy and lifelong single people, and the people who matter most to them, do not.

In Connecticut, Professor Geller discovered, farmers who are married couples (or people related by blood) can apply for "family farm" loans, but other farmers working cooperatively cannot. "What does marriage have to do with farming?" she asked.

In many universities, when a married candidate is offered a faculty position, special efforts are made to hire the spouse as well. "I had yet to hear a professor whose wife found work at his home institution ask why their marriage positively influenced hiring, when a candidate's maleness or heterosexuality could not," Professor Geller noted.

At college orientations and professional development programs, the value of diversity is touted. Yet, she found, "Marriage as a privileging category and relationship-status discrimination are largely ignored. One must wonder why seminars designed to highlight power imbalances don't question an institution that unequally distributes hundreds of benefits." In our personal correspondence, Professor Geller told me, "I've seen whole rooms full of academics armed with the customary terms—"privilege," "power," "hostility," "unsafe space,"—fall silent when I mention that I am paid a different salary than my colleagues, because I can't add another adult to my health plan."

Single people do not just miss out on the advantages accorded to married people just because they are married; they are also left mostly unprotected from discrimination. University of Virginia law professor Naomi Cahn noted that discrimination against singles "is not addressed by the major antidiscrimination federal laws,"[382] even when many other groups are explicitly protected. For example, the US Equal Employment Opportunity Commission warns that "It is illegal for an employer to discriminate against a job applicant because of his or her race, color, religion, sex (including gender identity, sexual orientation, and pregnancy), national origin, age (forty or older), disability, or genetic information."[383] Marital status is missing from that long list.

Before I started studying single life, I was oblivious to the many advantages bestowed by governments only on people who are legally married. Much more apparent to me—and to others as well—were the ways in which couples (and not just married couples) are recognized, respected, and celebrated in everyday life—as, for example, when events are organized and priced per couple, when friends and relatives ask after romantic partners but not best friends, and when romantic partners, but no one else, are deemed worthy of inclusion in extended-family vacations and reunions. People who are newly single after many years of marriage or committed coupling have told me that they are astounded by the differences in the ways they are treated. It works in the other direction too; people who have been single for a very long time, upon coupling, discover that they have suddenly gained entrée to a whole new world of inclusion, admiration, and respect. Coupling has become a prized and privileged status.

Angelica Malin, for example, has achieved more than she ever imagined. Her lifelong dream was to write a book—and now she has written three bestsellers. She has traveled globally as a professional public speaker and hosted conferences that have attracted thousands of participants. And yet, it was her announcement on social media of her whirlwind romance, culminating in marriage and a baby, that garnered warm congratulations from strangers as well as friends and family, stories in national newspapers, and TV appearances in two countries.[384]

Mini versions of Angelica's story play out every day on social media. Over the years, single people have told me that an announcement of a new romantic relationship—just an ordinary relationship, not some dramatic whirlwind story—brings a flood of likes and offerings of praise unlike anything they ever experience when posting about life achievements such as landing a new job, buying a home, or getting a degree.

Resistance to Noticing Singlism, or Acknowledging that There Is Anything Wrong with It

Here's an easy question. Suppose a landlord was choosing between two potential tenants, one black and the other white, and both had steady jobs and were described very positively by their current landlords. The black applicant offers to pay more than the white applicant, but you learn that "the landlord prefers to lease houses to white people and decides to accept the white person as the tenant." How would you explain that decision?

When Wendy Morris and Stacey Sinclair and I asked that question in our studies of housing discrimination, our participants answered just as we thought they would.[385] They said that the landlord was prejudiced and was basing the decision on stereotyping. We also asked them to rate how legitimate, justifiable, and reasonable they thought the decision was, and they rated it as very illegitimate, unjustifiable, and unreasonable.

We did four more versions of the same study, in which the landlord chose (1) a man over a woman even though the woman offered to pay more, or (2) a heterosexual over a lesbian or a gay person even though the latter offered to pay more, or (3) a thin person over a higher weight person even though the heavier person offered to pay more, or (4) a young person over an old person, even though the old person offered to pay more. In every instance, the prejudice and illegitimacy of the landlord's decision seemed self-evident to participants.

Then we did one more version, in which the landlord chose a married applicant over a single one, even though the single applicant offered to pay more. This time when we asked participants to explain the landlord's decision, only 10 percent said that the landlord was prejudiced. Instead, the most common answer was that the landlord chose the married couple "because they are married," and they didn't think there was anything wrong with that. They judged the landlord's decision to favor the married applicant as legitimate, justifiable, and reasonable—something that did not happen in any other versions of the study.

I think that kind of reasoning is shaped by the bedrock belief that coupling is natural and normal and superior to staying single. If single people really are inferior, what's the harm in treating them as such? They deserve it.

Also significant are the beliefs that single people don't like being single, that no one really wants to stay single, and—most importantly—that marital or romantic relationship status, unlike some other statuses, is something that can be changed. When I write about housing discrimination or any other examples of singlism on my blogs, someone predictably proposes what they see as a simple and fair solution: if single people want to be free from discrimination or if they want the legal benefits of marriage, then they should just get married. It's an insensitive suggestion, an affront to all the single people who would dearly love to marry and who have invested untold amounts of time and money into their attempts to do so, to no avail. And more to the point, no one should *have to* get married in order to be treated fairly.[386]

And yet the point is an important one. The perception of single status as something that can be changed, something that just about every single person *wants* to change, may well be one of the biggest obstacles to social justice and social change for people who are single. Why join a movement for singles' rights when single people will get all the benefits, privileges, and protections of coupling once they find that special someone?

People who are single at heart love being single and want to stay single. We have the potential to ignite a new social movement. I think it should be founded on our basic principles and values.

Principles and Values of the Single at Heart

The values of the single at heart are human values. Those values begin with the assumption that every human deserves the basics of a dignified life and build up to something even more ambitious—humans should be supported not just in their attempts to survive, but to flourish. Single at heart values recognize, fundamentally, that for some people, the path to flourishing is living single.

Single at heart values are inclusive and openhearted. People who are single at heart, like single people more generally as well as coupled people, come in many varieties, from many different backgrounds, and we value and respect them all.

We believe that all of the people who matter to us, and not just spouses or romantic partners, are deserving of recognition, respect, appreciation, and celebration. Acknowledging this is a call to support our interdependence and all of our caring relationships.

The single at heart value, rather than fear, the time and space they have to themselves. Acknowledging this is a call to support our independence and to encourage others to also appreciate solitude, solo pursuits, and private spaces.

Single at heart values bend the arc of the moral universe toward justice. In the long and noble tradition of challenging systems of inequality such as patriarchy and white supremacy that value some people more than others, our values challenge the presumed superiority of coupled people over single people.

1. **Basic human dignity**
   Everyone deserves the basics of human dignity. A person's value is not defined by their marital or romantic relationship status, and their rights, benefits, and protections should not be linked to those statuses either.

Everyone should have economic security: a living wage for those who can work, but also economic security that is not tied to employment, perhaps in the form of universal basic income. Everyone should also have the health care and the mental health care that they need, and educational opportunities too. Everyone should have clean water, good food, quality affordable housing, and personal safety. In their access to these basic components of human dignity, a person's marital or romantic relationship status should be completely irrelevant.

The possibilities for parenting should not depend on a person's marital or romantic relationship status either. Those include, for example, eligibility for adoption and access to assisted reproductive technologies and maternity or paternity benefits. Are you thinking that two-parent families should be prioritized over single-parent families in the adoption process, that those families would be better for the children? Just look back at what I've covered to remind yourself that single parents are not always raising their children single-handedly and that single-parent homes are often full of love and free of conflict between adults. Beware of being seduced by a belief in the Magical Mythical Romantic Partner.

The option not to parent should also be open to all. Whether a person can have birth control, sterilization, or an abortion should have nothing to do with their marital or romantic relationship status. It is not enough for the basic components of human dignity to be available; they also need to be accessible. In the United States, for example, some people have health insurance that covers certain procedures or surgeries, and yet they have trouble accessing those services. That can happen when hospitals require patients to have a ride back from a procedure from someone they know and not just a hired taxi or Uber driver, or when inpatients need another person present to help them or advocate for them, yet there are no options for patients who cannot easily meet those requirements.

If basic protections were extended to all people, no one would have to marry, or stay in a conflictual or even abusive marriage, just to get them. It would be a step toward dismantling systems of inequality.

2. **Valuing single life**
   Single life can be a happy, meaningful, and fulfilling life, not just for the moment, but for life. For the single at heart, it is not just a good life, it is the best life. Laws, policies, practices, and norms should be just as supportive of single people as coupled people.

Valuing single life just as much as coupled life would transform nearly every domain of life. I'll describe just a few examples.

If single people were valued, workplaces would be about work. No one would be paid any more or any less because of their marital status or romantic relationship status. Single people would not be required or pressured to subsidize their married coworkers—not with their money (as when married employees get benefits that they don't), not with their time (as when they are expected to put in more hours to cover for their coupled coworkers, or to work during holidays), and not with their gifts and emotions (as when employees are asked to cheer and celebrate the upcoming nuptials of their coworkers, but the achievements of their single coworkers are ignored).

If single life were valued, popular culture would feature more complex, compelling characters who are single at heart. There are a few here and there but identifying them is like playing *Where's Waldo?*—you have to look carefully and squint, and he'll still be very hard to find. It's not like finding the bride.

If single life were valued, young adults would be parented more effectively. Journalist Vicki Larson posed this question to parents of young adults who have always been single, aren't dating, and don't seem concerned about their single status: "What if our child announced that they were single at heart and would prefer platonic relationships—a.k.a. deep, meaningful friendships—over romantic ones?" She also offered an answer: "Can we just agree that we do nothing?"[387]

If single life were valued, single people would be more likely to be helped effectively when they seek psychotherapy. Some therapists seem to assume that the real problem troubling their single clients is that they are single, and the solution is to help them do the work it takes to successfully couple. In Israel, six married therapists working at a family therapy center compared notes about their treatment of their single clients, especially the single women. They were dismayed at what they discovered about themselves. As one said, "I thought it was my covert responsibility to get the woman to marry, even though I knew this was not my task as a therapist."[388]

The therapists decided to deprogram themselves. For eighteen months, they met every other week, spending two hours together each time. They compared notes on what their parents had said about marriage and about the single people they knew. They talked about different ways of thinking about singlehood. By the end, they resolved to listen to every single client with an open mind, so as "to enable her to choose a lifestyle and form an identity that is right for her, in accordance with her values and intentions."[389]

3. **Valuing all of the people who matter to us**

The people who matter to us are not defined by their marital or romantic relationship status. Laws, policies, practices, and norms should be supportive of all the important people in our lives. Caring relationships and communities of care should be supported regardless of the marital, romantic relationship, parental, or family status of the people receiving or providing care.

If friends and other people who are important to us were taken more seriously, all of our lives would be transformed for the better. A variety of creative living arrangements would be available, with more dreamed up all the time. Remember the Golden Girls? They would no longer be just fictional characters. Real people too, who preferred not to live alone, would look to friends and relatives as a matter of course; they would be relieved of the pressure to couple, recouple, or stay coupled as their only option short of seeking roommates they don't even know.

Remember those seven women from China (from Chapter 3, "Freedom") who did not wait until they were old to build the house of their fantasies and share their lives there? Instead of being one of those stories that goes viral because it is so unique, it would be one of many examples of people building their lives around their friends rather than spouses or romantic partners.

In some places, laws and policies would need to be changed to support a greater variety of living arrangements. For example, zoning laws that bar a certain number of unrelated adults from sharing a home could, if left on the books, turn the Golden Girls into criminals.

If all of the important people in our lives were valued, I think child-rearing would be transformed too. I am an enthusiastic supporter of single people who want to raise children in places of their own, with no other adults under the same roof and no one else with decision-making powers over their children. But I also understand that many people (and not just women) yearn to be parents, yet do not want to parent on their own. They think that a committed romantic partner is their only real option, and they fear that not finding such a person spells the end of their dream of raising children. Maybe they have never heard of resources such as Modamily.com, a platform that has been helping people find platonic co-parents (and sperm donors) since 2011. But parenting with strangers or giving up on the possibility of parenting would not be the only options if we took relationships other than romantic ones more seriously. Imagine if it became commonplace to raise children with friends, relatives, or other people who are already known and trusted, or if the stories of people who have already done so became more widely known and celebrated.[390]

Finding friends, and maybe even keeping them, would be easier if we valued friends more. Matchmaking would be liberated from its tired old erotic box, and people would be more mindful and more intentional about introducing potential friends. Online platforms and apps would more often cater to friend-finders and not just date-seekers. The plus-one on invitations would be routinely understood to include friends and not just romantic partners. People would less often demote their friends upon coupling, because they would understand what they are missing. Single and coupled people would celebrate the anniversaries of their friendships. Political candidates would boast about their friends and have them at their sides at key moments. Friends would more often be named as beneficiaries. Moving to live near a friend would be unremarkable, and employers would understand that their employees may be reluctant to relocate if it meant leaving cherished friends behind. Paid leave to care for close friends, as well as bereavement leave to mourn them, would not be at the discretion of employers—it would be the law.

If workplaces offer married workers the option to add their spouse to their health care plans at a reduced rate, then single workers too should have the option to add a person who is important to them to their plans. The same is true for any other benefits or perks extended to spouses or romantic partners. Either all workers get the benefit, or none do. An alternative system that would also be fair is one in which all workers are allotted the same amount of money, with the option to spend it on whichever available benefits they choose.

Recognizing and valuing the important people in our lives is not just a matter of fairness. Sometimes our very survival is at stake. When Joan DelFattore was diagnosed with Stage 4 gallbladder cancer, her oncologist asked if she had a husband or other immediate family members. She didn't, and he interrupted her when she tried to tell him about her devoted circle of friends. Then he recommended the less aggressive treatment, telling her he wouldn't risk the serious side effects of the more effective one with "someone in your situation."[391]

She found a different oncologist who did listen, then years later, made it her mission to find out whether the first doctor's bias was widespread. She reviewed eighty-four studies from a National Cancer Institute database that tracks millions of cancer patients. Her conclusion, published in the *New England Journal of Medicine*, states: " . . . this body of medical literature overwhelmingly equates the absence of a spouse with a lack of social support."[392] Too many oncologists believe that people who don't have a spouse don't have anyone, and then go on to recommend suboptimal treatments. Professor DelFattore's article was published under the title, "Death by stereotype?"

4. **Valuing solitude**
   The ability to spend some time alone comfortably is valuable to individuals and society. Choosing to do so should be respected and supported; living alone should be too.

For individuals, spending time alone for positive reasons has scientifically proven psychological benefits. At the societal level, loneliness would be less rampant if people were less fearful of solitude and more adept at tapping into its potential.

If solitude were valued, parents and teachers would be just as concerned about children having trouble spending time on their own as they are with children having trouble making friends. They would feel proud of the children (and adults) who flourish in solitude, and they would learn how to teach relevant skills to those who don't.

If solitude were valued, living alone would be valued and supported too. Appropriate housing would be plentiful and affordable. More apartments and homes would be designed or adapted to make solo living safer and easier for people with disabilities and other people who may need adaptations as they age.

Products such as perishable foods would be sold in small portions (without being priced disproportionately higher). Platforms for finding help with tasks that can be difficult to handle alone, such as Angi and Thumbtack, would be available in more places. Community-based helping would also be encouraged. In Buy Nothing groups, for example, members give away items they don't want, or offer their expertise, for free; members can also ask for what they need and owe nothing except perhaps a word of thanks.

> In a culture in which interpersonal relationships are generally considered to be the answer to every form of distress, it is sometimes difficult to persuade well-meaning helpers that solitude can be as therapeutic as emotional support.[393] —Anthony Storr, *Solitude: A Return to Self*

Of all the kinds of professional helpers who are tasked with working with older people, those who are specifically trained to do so, such as gerontologists, should be among the most insightful. They should understand, for example, the kinds of experiences that older people enjoy.

In Israel, three gerontology researchers asked gerontology occupational therapists and gerontology graduate students whether they thought that, for older people, spending time by themselves could be a positive experience.[394] Seventeen percent of the graduate students said no. All of the occupational therapists understood that older people can enjoy being by themselves, but they qualified their answers, saying, for example, that solitude would only be agreeable for older people who have rich inner lives or for those who are healthy.

The researchers also asked dozens of older people, between the ages of sixty-five and 103, the same question: "Can being by oneself be a positive or agreeable experience?" All of them said yes, and none of them qualified their answers. As examples, they described how much they enjoyed their solitude while fishing, making coffee, appreciating art, reminiscing, and training for triathlons.

If solitude were valued and understood, older people would be treated more effectively and more appropriately. I live alone, but maybe someday that will no longer be possible. I'm dismayed by the prospect of well-meaning professionals trying to coax me into doing activities because they don't believe that I could enjoy time to myself.

5. **Valuing our differences**

   People who are single at heart, like other single people and like coupled people, are very diverse. Those differences should be acknowledged and respected. The single at heart should not be stereotyped or caricatured.

People who are single at heart share a love of single life, solitude, and freedom. Beyond that, we vary tremendously. We differ, for example, in the number and kinds of people we want in our life, in what intimacy means to us, and in the mix of time alone and time with other people we find optimal. We vary greatly in our interests and passions, in our financial resources, and in the kinds of living arrangements we like best.

In the realm of housing, for example, it is sometimes assumed that appropriate dwellings for people who live alone would be tiny apartments or homes. For some single people, that is their preference, and for others, it is all they can afford. But other single people want and can afford larger places, and those preferences should be acknowledged just as readily as the same preferences expressed by couples. They aren't always. When I expressed an interest in seeing a three-bedroom home that was available to rent, the owner refused to show it to me until I explained why a single woman would need three bedrooms. (I didn't bother.)

Innovative housing arrangements are of great interest to people who want easy access to both privacy and companionship. Cohousing communities, for example, include private homes, often arranged around open green spaces, along with a "common house" where community members can share meals, convene meetings, or pursue other interests, such as artwork or exercising, in spaces designed for those purposes. In other kinds of arrangements, people all live under the same roof in one big house, but have rooms or suites of their own, sometimes with separate entrances.[395]

6. **Beyond the basics: the opportunity to flourish**
   Individuals and societies flourish when people are free to pursue their most meaningful, fulfilling, and psychologically rich lives. Pursuits other than coupling that provide meaning, fulfillment, and psychological richness should be supported just as much as coupling.

In the workplace, time off should not be limited to new parents and other caregivers, or to those who need medical or bereavement leave. Opportunities for personal development should be available too.

In everyday life, the achievements and milestones that single people find meaningful and fulfilling should be acknowledged and celebrated. They might include, for example, landing a coveted job, leaving an awful one, graduating, moving to a new place, buying a home, marking twenty-five years of friendship, completing a creative project, and running a marathon.

Fostering opportunities for single people to flourish should be on the global agenda. As Sasha Roseneil, lead author of *The Tenacity of the Couple-Norm*, wrote in an op-ed, we need to "start thinking about how international human rights conventions might be extended to place the right to a fulfilling single life alongside the right to family life."[396]

Into the Future

The right to be oneself—on one's own terms and with whomever one chooses—is itself a fundamental form of individual liberty.[397]
—Catherine Powell, "Up from Marriage: Freedom, Solitude,
and Individual Autonomy in the Shadow of Marriage Equality"

My mission in putting the single at heart on the map is to rewrite what it means to be single. Single life, to those of us who are single at heart, is a joyful place, a place to learn and grow. It is a big-hearted, expansive, meaningful life full of possibilities. We love and care for people beyond just romantic partners and are loved and cared for in return. Intimacy, to us, is personal; in that domain as in all others, we follow our hearts rather than the cultural rulebooks. We chart our own life courses, with meaningfulness, psychological richness, and authenticity as our guides.

A new and more enlightened understanding of what it can mean to be single—and to be human—would of course be a tremendous boon to people who are single at heart. We've been doubted and disparaged for so long; it would be sublime to be validated and appreciated instead.

Those of us who already understand ourselves as single at heart are not the only ones who would benefit. So too would all those children, teens, and young adults still trying to get to know themselves. A new option would be available to them, as liberating and as meaningful as the realization that not everyone is heterosexual. It would also be freeing to adults of all ages who are teetering on the edge of claiming single life, but reluctant to take the leap.

Marriage rates would probably decline. Fewer new romantic relationships would be launched. But that too would be a good thing, because the people drawn to such partnerships would be those who really want them. They will be free to find someone who really does want a conventionally coupled life. Parents will be freed from the worrying assumption that there is something amiss about their grown single kids. Mothers on their deathbeds will tell their single at heart adult children how very proud they are that their children are living their best, most authentic lives.

NOTES

1 Tetyana Pudrovska, Scott Schieman, and Deborah Carr, "Strains of Singlehood in Later Life: Do Race and Gender Matter?" *The Journals of Gerontology: Series B* 61, no. 6 (2006): S315–S322.

2 Julie Cwikel, Helen Gramotnev, and Christina Lee, "Never-married childless women in Australia: Health and social circumstances in older age," *Social Science & Medicine* 62, no. 8 (2006) 1991–2001.

3 Elyakim Kislev, "Reduced Relationship Desire Is Associated with Better Life Satisfaction for Singles in Germany: An Analysis of Pairfam Data," *Journal of Social and Personal Relationships* 38, no. 7 (2021): 2073–2083.

4 Elyakim Kislev, "How Do Relationship Desire and Sociability Relate to Each Other Among Singles? Longitudinal Analysis of the Pairfam Survey," *Journal of Social and Personal Relationships* 37, no. 8–9 (2020): 2634–2650.

5 Elyakim Kislev, "The Sexual Activity and Sexual Satisfaction of Singles in the Second Demographic Transition," *Sexuality Research and Social Policy* 18 (2021): 726–738.

6 Daniel Victor, "A Pandemic Is Hard Enough. For Some, Being Single Has Made It Harder," *New York Times,* January 29, 2021, https://www.nytimes.com/2021/01/29/style/single-people-covid.html.

7 ClinOncDoc, December 19, 2020, 4:26 p.m., https://twitter.com/ClinOncDoc/status/1340408303592026112.

8 Bella DePaulo, "Covid Singles Are Supposedly Lonely and Miserable. But Some of Us Are Thriving Instead," *NBC Think,* March 13, 2021, https://www.nbcnews.com/think/opinion/covid-singles-are-supposedly-lonely-miserable-some-us-are-thriving-ncna1261021.

9 Bella DePaulo, "How the Pandemic Created a Cohort of Secure Single People," Psychology Today, April 1, 2021, https://www.psychologytoday.com/us/blog/living-single/202104/how-the-pandemic-created-cohort-secure-single-people.

10 Bella DePaulo, "Single in a Pandemic: 18 Reflections at the 1-Year Mark." Medium, April 2, 2021, https://belladepaulo.medium.com/single-in-a-pandemic-18-reflections-at-the-1-year-mark-6099a4bf365.

11 Emma Ailes, "'Covid Ended Our Marriage': The Couples Who Split in the Pandemic," BBC World Service, December 3, 2020, https://www.bbc.com/news/world-55146909.

12 Dave McGinn, "Alone Time Becomes Car Time: Finding Moments of Solitude May Help Ease Pandemic Stress," *Globe and Mail,* April 4, 2021, https://www.theglobeandmail.com/life/health-and-fitness/article-alone-time-becomes-car-time-finding-moments-of-solitude-may-help-ease/.

13 Erika Mailman, "The Rise of the Pandemic Shed," *Washington Post,* April 5, 2021, https://www.washingtonpost.com/magazine/2021/04/05/shed-plans-pandemic-families/?itid=hp-top-table-main.

14 Katie Van Syckle, "A Window into a Changed America," *New York Times,* April 17, 2021, https://www.nytimes.com/2021/04/17/insider/pandemic-life-transformations.html.

15 United Nations, "World Population Prospects 2022: Summary of Results," July 2022, https://www.un.org/development/desa/pd/sites/www.un.org.development.desa.pd/files/undesa_pd_2022_wpp_key-messages.pdf.

16 Esteban Ortiz-Ospina, "The Rise of Living Alone: How One-Person Households Are Becoming Increasingly Common Around the World," *Our World in Data,* December 10, 2019, https://ourworldindata.org/living-alone.

17 OECD Family Database, "Family Size and Household Composition," Table SF1.1.A. Types of Household, 2011, updated June 12, 2016, https://www.oecd.org/els/family/SF_1_1_Family_size_and_composition.pdf.

18 United Nations Women, "Progress of the World's Women 2019-2022: Families in a Changing World," https://www.unwomen.org/en/digital-library/progress-of-the-worlds-women.

19 OECD Family Database, "Marriage and Divorce Rates," Chart SF3.1.A. Crude Marriage Rate, 1970, 1995, 2019 and 2020 or Latest Available Year. Updated June 2022.

20 R. Kelly Raley and Megan M. Sweeney, "Divorce, Repartnering, and Stepfamilies: A Decade in Review," *Journal of Marriage and Family* 82, no. 1 (2020): 81–99.

21 Ibid.

22 Bella DePaulo, *Singled Out: How Singles Are Stereotyped, Stigmatized, and Ignored, and Still*

Live Happily Ever After (New York: St. Martin's Griffin, 2007).

23 Eli J. Finkel, Chin Ming Hui, Kathleen L. Carswell, and Grace M. Larson, "The Suffocation of Marriage: Climbing Mount Maslow Without Enough Oxygen," *Psychological Inquiry* 25, no. 1 (2014): 1–41.

24 Tara Parker-Pope, "Normal Marital Hatred Is Real. Here's What to Do about It," *Washington Post*, September 23, 2022, https://www.washingtonpost.com/wellness/2022/09/23/marriage-relationships-conflict/.

25 Joseph Chamie, "Out-of-Wedlock Births Rise Worldwide," YaleGlobal Online, March 16, 2017, https://archive-yaleglobal.yale.edu/content/out-wedlock-births-rise-worldwide.

26 United Nations Women, "Progress of the World's Women 2019–2022: Families in a Changing World."

27 Kim Parker and Wendy Wang, "Record Share of Americans Have Never Married," Pew Research Center, September 24, 2014, https://www.pewresearch.org/social-trends/2014/09/24/record-share-of-americans-have-never-married/.

28 US Census Bureau, "Table A1. America's Families and Living Arrangements: 2021," *Marital Status of People 15 Years and Over, by Age, Sex, and Personal Earnings: 2021*, https://www.census.gov/data/tables/2021/demo/families/cps-2021.html.

29 Anna Brown, "A Profile of Single Americans," Pew Research Center. August 20, 2020. https://www.pewresearch.org/social-trends/2020/08/20/a-profile-of-single-americans/.

30 Anna Brown, "Nearly Half of US Adults Say Dating Has Gotten Harder for Most People in the Last 10 Years," Pew Research Center. August 20, 2020. https://www.pewresearch.org/social-trends/2020/08/20/nearly-half-of-u-s-adults-say-dating-has-gotten-harder-for-most-people-in-the-last-10-years/.

31 Anna Brown, "Most Americans Who Are 'Single and Looking' Say Dating Has Been Harder During the Pandemic," Pew Research Center. April 6, 2022. https://www.pewresearch.org/fact-tank/2022/04/06/most-americans-who-are-single-and-looking-say-dating-has-been-harder-during-the-pandemic/.

32 Selby Fleming McPhee, "Once More unto the Breach," *Vassar Quarterly*, Spring/Summer 2017.

33 William J. Scarborough, Joanna R. Pepin, Danny L. Lambouths III, Ronald Kwon, and Ronaldo Monasterio, "The Intersection of Racial and Gender Attitudes, 1977 through 2018," *American Sociological Review* 85, no. 5 (2021): 823–855.

34 Ibid.

35 Phrases such as "racialized as black" or "racialized as white" are sometimes used instead of "black" or "white" to suggest a less essentialist or biological understanding of race; D.T. Williams, "Racism and the Mechanisms Maintaining Racial Stratification in Black Families." *Journal of Family Theory and Review*, 2023.

36 US Government Accountability Office, *Defense of Marriage Act: Update to Prior Report*, 2004, https://www.gao.gov/products/gao-04-353r.

37 Betty Friedan, *The Feminine Mystique* (New York: W.W. Norton, 1963/2001), 82.

38 Sasha Roseneil, Isabel Crowhurst, Tone Hellesund, Ana Cristina Santos, and Mariya Stoilova, *The Tenacity of the Couple-Norm: Intimate Citizen Regimes in a Changing Europe* (London: UCL Press, 2020).

39 Ibid.

40 Carolyn Hax, "Carolyn Hax Chat," Happy Singleness. *Washington Post*, July 9, 2021. https://www.washingtonpost.com/lifestyle/2021/07/09/live-chat-carolyn-hax/.

41 Ibid.

42 Hill Holiday, "The 'Shunned' Single Woman," June 14, 2018. https://www.businesswire.com/news/home/20180614005260/en/.

43 Kislev, "How Do Relationship Desire and Sociability Relate to Each Other Among Singles?" 2634–2650.

44 Bella M. DePaulo and Wendy L. Morris, "Singles in Society and in Science," *Psychological Inquiry* 16, no. 1–2 (2005): 57–83.

45 Kislev, "Reduced Relationship Desire Is Associated with Better Life Satisfaction for Singles in Germany: An Analysis of Pairfam Data," 2073–2083.

46 Karen Gail Lewis, "Being Single Is an Ambiguous Loss," N.d., accessed January 13, 2023. https://drkarengaillewis.com/articles-being-single-is-an-ambiguous-loss.

47 Lori Gottlieb, "Dear Therapist: It's Hard to Accept Being Single," *The Atlantic*, June 3, 2019. https://www.theatlantic.com/family/archive/2019/06/how-be-okay-being-single/590854/.

48 Stephanie S. Spielmann, Geoff MacDonald, Jessica A. Maxwell, Samantha Joel, Diana

Peragine, Amy Muise, and Emily A. Impett, "Settling for Less Out of Fear of Being Single," *Journal of Personality and Social Psychology* 105, no. 6 (2013): 1049–1073.

49 Ibid.

50 Stephanie S. Spielmann, Geoff MacDonald, Samantha Joel, and Emily A. Impett, "Longing for Ex-Partners Out of Fear of Being Single," *Journal of Personality* 84, no. 6 (2016): 799–808.

51 Laura Kipnis, *Against Love: A Polemic* (New York: Vintage, 2004), 84.

52 Nathan W. Hudson, Richard E. Lucas, and M. Brent Donnellan, "The Highs and Lows of Love: Romantic Relationship Quality Moderates Whether Spending Time with One's Partner Predicts Gains or Losses in Well-Being," *Personality and Social Psychology Bulletin* 46, no. 4 (2020): 572–589.

53 Janesha Jones, "Tracee Ellis Ross Responds to Being the 'Poster Child for Being Single,'" *Atlanta Black Star*, October 28, 2021, https://atlantablackstar.com/2021/10/28/tracee-ellis-ross-responds-to-being-the-poster-child-for-being-single/.

54 Shigehiro Oishi and Erin C. Westgate, "A Psychologically Rich Life: Beyond Happiness and Meaning," *Psychological Review* 129, no. 4 (2022): 790–811.

55 Ibid, 790.

56 Ibid, 792.

57 Nadine F. Marks and James David Lambert, "Marital Status Continuity and Change Among Young and Midlife Adults," *Journal of Family Issues* 19, no. 6 (1998): 652–686.

58 Oishi and Westgate, "A Psychologically Rich Life: Beyond Happiness and Meaning," 799.

59 Richard M. Ryan and Edward L. Deci, "Self-Determination Theory and the Facilitation of Intrinsic Motivation, Social Development, and Well-Being," *American Psychologist* 55, no. 1 (2000): 68–78.

60 Kristen M. Bernhardt, "Party of One: Legitimizing Single and Solo Life through Personal Narratives," master's thesis, New Mexico State University, 2017.

61 Elizabeth Brake, *Minimizing Marriage: Marriage, Morality, and the Law* (New York: Oxford University Press, 2012), 88–89.

62 Hattie Crisell, "The Rise of the Alpha Single," *Times* magazine, March 17, 2018, https://www.thetimes.co.uk/article/the-rise-of-the-alpha-single-spk8s73q8.

63 Vera Moore, "I Stopped Dating and I Couldn't Be Happier," Medium, January 28, 2022, https://medium.com/fourth-wave/i-stopped-dating-and-couldnt-be-happier-a24226074d2e.

64 Leon H. Vincent, "A Successful Bachelor," *Atlantic Monthly*, January 28, 2022, https://www.theatlantic.com/magazine/archive/1898/06/a-successful-bachelor/306487/.

65 Ibid.

66 Ibid.

67 Ibid.

68 Ibid.

69 Ibid.

70 Bella DePaulo, "Single, Married, Living Alone: 10 Ways Men and Women Differ," *Psychology Today*, August 1, 2020, https://www.psychologytoday.com/us/blog/living-single/202008/single-married-living-alone-10-ways-men-and-women-differ.

71 Maike Luhmann, Wilhelm Hofmann, Michael Eid, and Richard E. Lucas, "Subjective Well-Being and Adaptation to Life Events: A Meta-Analysis," *Journal of Personality and Social Psychology* 102, no. 3 (2012): 592–615.

72 DePaulo, "Single, Married, Living Alone: 10 Ways Men and Women Differ." *Psychology Today* (blog), August 1, 2020, https://www.psychologytoday.com/us/blog/living-single/202008/single-married-living-alone-10-ways-men-and-women-differ.

73 Margaret F. Brinig and Douglas W. Allen, "These Boots Are Made for Walking: Why Most Divorce Filers Are Women," *American Law and Economics Review* 2, no. 1 (2000): 126–169.

74 Raley and Sweeney, "Divorce, Repartnering, and Stepfamilies: A Decade in Review," 81–99.

75 Janelle Jones, "5 Facts About the State of the Gender Pay Gap," US Department of Labor Blog, March 19, 2021, https://blog.dol.gov/2021/03/19/5-facts-about-the-state-of-the-gender-pay-gap.

76 Dimitri Mortelmans, "Economic Consequences of Divorce: A Review," *Parental Life Courses after Separation and Divorce in Europe*, edited by Michaela Kreyenfeld and Heike Trappe, 23–41 (Cham, Switzerland: Springer Open).

77 Fenaba R. Addo and Daniel T. Lichter, "Marriage, Marital History, and Black—White Wealth Differentials Among Older Women," *Journal of Marriage and Family* 75, no. 2 (2013): 342–362.

78 Susan Sprecher and Diane Felmlee, "Social Network Pressure on Women and Men to En-

ter a Romantic Relationship and Fear of Being Single," *Interpersona* 15, no. 2 (2021): 246–261.

79 Lucas Bradley, "Single Manhood Is So Much More Than the Stereotypes," *Psychology Today*, January 3, 2022, https://www.psychologyto-day.com/us/blog/living-single/202201/single-manhood-is-so-much-more-the-stereotypes.

80 Ketaki Chowkhani and Craig Wynne, eds. *Singular Selves: An Introduction to Singles Studies* (New York: Routledge, 2023).

81 Craig Wynne, *How to Be a Happy Bachelor* (Dubuque, IA: Kendall Hunt Publishing, 2020).

82 Nancy Waithira, "What Happens to Men Who Stay Bachelors for a Lifetime?" *Nation.Africa*, November 27, 2021, https://nation.africa/ken-ya/life-and-style/saturday-magazine/what-happens-to-men-who-stay-bachelors-for-a-lifetime--3632370.

83 Justin A. Lavner, Benjamin R. Karney, and Thomas N. Bradbury, "Do Cold Feet Warn of Trouble Ahead? Premarital Uncertainty and Four-Year Marital Outcomes," *Journal of Family Psychology* 26, no. 6 (2012): 1012–1017.

84 Bibi Dietz, "How to Tell If You're Meant to Stay Single." *Bustle*, March 16, 2016, https://www.bustle.com/articles/145642-were-you-meant-to-stay-single-15-ways-to-know.

85 US Census Bureau, Table MS-2, "Estimated Median Age at First Marriage, by Sex: 1890 to the Present," US Census Bureau, Decennial Censuses, 1890 to 1940, and Current Population Survey, March, and Annual Social and Economic Supplements, 1947 to 2022, https://www.census.gov/data/tables/time-series/demo/families/marital.html.

86 A. Böger, and O. Huxhold, "The changing relationship between partnership status and loneliness: Effects related to aging and historical time." *The Journals of Gerontology: Series B: Psychological Sciences and Social Sciences*, 75 (7), 1423–1432, https://doi.org/10.1093/geronb/gby153.

87 Joan DelFattore, "Why I'm Single: Then and Now," *Psychology Today*, November 12, 2016, https://www.psychologytoday.com/us/blog/living-single/201611/why-i-m-single-then-and-now.

88 K. Chowkhani, "Singlehood Unlimited: Solo Living in South India," *Unattached: Essays on Singlehood*, edited by Angelica Malin (London: Square Peg, 2022) 54–58.

89 The Community of Single People includes some members who are not single at heart. A newer Facebook group, Single People at Heart, includes only people who are single at heart.

90 Christina Patterson, *The Art of Not Falling Apart: A Shockingly Honest Celebration of Life as an Adventure.* (London: Atlantic Books, 2018).

91 Kris Marsh, *The Love Jones Cohort: Single and Living Alone in the Black Middle Class* (Cambridge: Cambridge University Press, 2023).

92 Carly Ledbetter, "Allison Janney Opens Up About Why She Never Married or Had Kids," HuffPost, April 7, 2021, https://www.huff-post.com/entry/allison-janney-why-she-nev-er-married-had-children_n_606db7f-5c5b68ddf94b79642.

93 Elyakim Kislev, "Happiness, Post-Materialistic Values, and the Unmarried," *Journal of Happiness Studies* 19, no. 8 (2018): 2243–2265.

94 Ed Anderson, "Savor the Freedom," *Good Bachelorhood*, February 24, 2022. https://goodbachelorhood.com/savor-the-freedom/.

95 Jamila Bookwala and Erin Fekete, "The Role of Psychological Resources in the Affective Well-Being of Never-Married Adults," *Journal of Social and Personal Relationships* 26, no. 4 (2009): 411–428.

96 Havighurst, Robert. *Human Development and Education* (Harlow, UK: Longmans, Green, 1953).

97 Juliana Menasce Horowitz, Nikki Graf, and Gretchen Livingston, "Marriage and Cohabitation in the US," Pew Research Center, November 6, 2019, https://www.pewresearch.org/social-trends/2019/11/06/marriage-and-co-habitation-in-the-u-s/.

98 Lisa Arnold and Christina Campbell, "The High Price of Being Single in America," *The Atlantic*, January 14, 2013, https://www.theat-lantic.com/sexes/archive/2013/01/the-high-price-of-being-single-in-america/267043/.

99 Elizabeth H Gorman, "Marriage and Money: The Effect of Marital Status on Attitudes Toward Pay and Finances," *Work and Occupations* 27, no. 1 (2000): 64–78.

100 Monica Kirpatrick Johnson, "Family Roles and Work Values: Processes of Selection and Change," *Journal of Marriage and Family* 67, no. 2 (2005): 352–369.

101 Elyakim Kislev, *Happy Singlehood: The Rising Acceptance and Celebration of Solo Living* (Oakland, CA: University of California Press, 2019).

102 Krista Tippett, host, "Sandra Cisneros: A House of Her Own," On Being (podcast), Feb-

ruary 13, 2020, https://onbeing.org/programs/sandra-cisneros-a-house-of-her-own/.

103 Keturah Kendrick, "Unmarried and Unbothered: Black Women Who Prefer Autonomy Over Marriage," *Black Ballad*, September 6, 2021, https://blackballad.co.uk/views-voices/unmarried-unbothered-black-women-who-prefer-autonomy-over-marriage.

104 Kislev, *Happy Singlehood*, 60.

105 US Bureau of Labor Statistics, "Table 4: Volunteers by Type of Main Organization for Which Volunteers Activities Were Performed and Selected Characteristics, September 2015," https://www.bls.gov/news.release/volun.t04.htm#.

106 Joan R. Kahn, Brittany S. McGill, and Suzanne M. Bianchi, "Help to Family and Friends: Are There Gender Differences at Older Ages?" *Journal of Marriage and Family*, 73, no. 1 (2011): 77–92.

107 Eric. Klinenberg, *Going Solo: The Extraordinary Rise and Surprising Appeal of Living Alone* (New York: Penguin Press, 2012).

108 James N. Laditka and Sarah B. Laditka, "Adult Children Helping Older Parents: Variations in Likelihood and Hours by Gender, Race, and Family Role," *Research on Aging 23*, no. 4 (2001): 429–456.

109 Ursula Henz, "Informal Caregiving at Working Age: Effects of Job Characteristics and Family Configuration," *Journal of Marriage and Family* 68, no. 2 (2006): 411–429.

110 Marsh, *The Love Jones Cohort*, 104–105.

111 Virpi Timonen and Martha Doyle, "Life-Long Singlehood: Intersections of the Past and Present," *Ageing & Society* 34, no. 10 (2014): 1749–1770.

112 Santos, Henri C., Michael E. W. Varnum, and Igor Grossman, "Global Increases in Individualism," *Psychological Science* 28, no. 9 (2017): 1228–1239.

113 Christine Emba, "Liberalism Is Loneliness," *Washington Post*, April 6, 2018, https://www.washingtonpost.com/opinions/liberalism-is-loneliness/2018/04/06/02a01aec-39ce-11e8-8fd2-49fe3c675a89_story.html.

114 Shawn A. Rhoads, Devon Gunter, Rebecca M. Ryan, and Abigail A. Marsh, "Global Variation in Subjective Well-Being Predicts Seven Forms of Altruism," *Psychological Science* 32, no. 8 (2021): 1247–1261.

115 Abigail Marsh, "Everyone Thinks Americans Are Selfish. They're Wrong," *New York Times*, May 26, 2021, https://www.nytimes.com/2021/05/26/opinion/individualism-united-states-altruism.html.

116 Eleanor Wilkinson, "Single People's Geographies of Home: Intimacy and Friendship Beyond 'the Family'," *Environment and Planning A: Economy and Space* 46, no. 10 (2014): 2452–2468.

117 Christopher Cameron, "Seven Chinese Girlfriends Buy Mansion to Retire and Die Together," *New York Post*, July 3, 2019, https://nypost.com/2019/07/03/seven-chinese-girlfriends-buy-mansion-to-retire-and-die-together/.

118 Steven Bereznai, *Gay and Single . . . Forever?* (New York: Marlowe & Company, 2006), 172.

119 Cristina Campbell, "Sitting on the Couch in Stained Sweatpants: Is It Cool?" *Onely*, July 13, 2020. https://onely.org/2020/07/13/sitting-on-the-couch-in-stained-sweatpants-is-it-cool/.

120 bell hooks, "Marginality as a Site of Resistance," in *Out There: Marginality and Contemporary Culture*, eds. Russell Ferguson, Martha Gever, Trinh T. Minh-ha, and Cornel West, (Cambridge, MA: MIT Press, 1992) 341–343.

121 Jill Summerville, "Single Women with Disabilities, Part 1: Guest Post by Jill Summerville," *Unmarried Equality*, February 26, 2022, https://www.unmarried.org/featured/single-women-with-disabilities-part-1-guest-post-by-jill-summerville/.

122 Chalandra M. Bryant, "African American Fictive Kin: Historical and Contemporary Notions," *Family Focus: Fictive Kin*, National Council on Family Relations, Spring 2018.

123 Kim TallBear, "Making Love and Relations: Beyond Settler Sex and Family," in *Queerly Canadian: An Introductory Reader in Sexuality Studies*, 2nd ed., eds. Scott Rayter and Laine Halpern Zisman (Toronto, Ontario: Women's Press, 2022).

124 Marsh, *The Love Jones Cohort*.

125 Bama, "Uphill flows the river," *Single by choice: Happily unmarried women!* Ed. K. Sharma, (New Delhi: Women Unlimited. 2019), 51–63.

126 Ibid, 54–55.

127 Fenton Johnson, *At the Center of All Beauty: Solitude and the Creative Life* (New York: W.W. Norton, 2020), 3.

128 Ibid, 9.

129 DePaulo and Morris, "Singles in Society and in Science," 57–83.

130 May Sarton, *Mrs. Stevens Hears the Mermaids Singing* (New York: Open Road Media, 2014 edition), 92.

131 Alice Koller, *The Stations of Solitude* (New York: Bantam Books, 1991), 4.

132 Anna Quinn, "Maybe," *Alone Together: Love, Grief, and Comfort in the Time of COVID-19*, ed. Jennifer Haupt, (Delta, British Columbia: Central Avenue Publishing, 2020), 94.

133 Virginia Thomas and Margarita Azmitia, "Motivation Matters: Development and Validation of the Motivation for Solitude Scale – Short Form (MSS-SF)," *Journal of Adolescence* 70, no. 1 (2019): 33–42.

134 Thuy-vy Nguyen, Richard M. Ryan, and Edward L. Deci, "Solitude as an Approach to Affective Self-Regulation," *Personality and Social Psychology Bulletin* 44, no. 1 (2018): 92–106.

135 Thuy-vy Nguyen, Netta Weinstein, and Richard M. Ryan, "The Possibilities of Aloneness and Solitude: Developing an Understanding Framed Through the Lens of Human Motivation and Needs," *The Handbook of Solitude: Psychological Perspectives on Social Isolatoin, Social Withdrawal, and Being Alone*, 2nd ed., eds. Robert J. Coplan, Julie C. Bowker, and Larry J. Nelson, (New York: Wiley-Blackwell, 2021), 224–239.

136 Stephanie Rosenbloom, *Alone Time: Four Seasons, Four Cities, and the Pleasures of Solitude* (New York: Viking, 2018), 38.

137 Johnson, *At the Center of All Beauty*, 65.

138 Sara Maitland, *How to Be Alone* (New York: Picador, 2014), 186.

139 Nguyen et al., "The Possibilities of Aloneness and Solitude: Developing an Understanding Framed Through the Lens of Human Motivation and Needs."

140 Chelom E. Leavitt, Bethany Butzer, Rebecca Clarke, and Kami Dvorakova, "Intentional Solitude and Mindfulness: The Benefits of Being Alone," *The Handbook of Solitude: Psychological Perspectives on Social Isolatoin, Social Withdrawal, and Being Alone*, 2nd ed., ed. Robert J. Coplan, Julie C. Bowker, and Larry J. Nelson (New York: Wiley-Blackwell, 2021), 340–350.

141 Maitland, *How to Be Alone*, 80.

142 Yuval Palgi, Dikla Segel-Karpas, Sharon Ost Mor, Yaakov Hoffman, Amit Shrira, and Ehud Bodner, "Positive Solitude Scale: Theoretical Background, Development and Validation," *Journal of Happiness Studies* 22, no. 8 (2021): 3357–3384.

143 Angela Haupt, "13 books to help you weather the rest of 2020 and beyond." *Washington Post*, October 5, 2020, https://www.washingtonpost.com/road-to-recovery/13-books-to-help-you-weather-the-rest-of-2020-and-beyond/2020/10/05/e5398bca-0714-11eb-9be6-cf25fb429f1a_story.html.

144 Nguyen et al., "The Possibilities of Aloneness and Solitude: Developing an Understanding Framed Through the Lens of Human Motivation and Needs," 224–239.

145 Ibid.

146 Ibid.

147 Nguyen, "Time Alone (Chosen or Not) Can Be a Chance to Hit the Reset Button."

148 Maitland, *How to Be Alone*, 21.

149 Anneli Rufus, *Party of One: The Loners' Manifesto* (Philadelphia: Da Capo Press, 2003).

150 Liad Uziel, "Alone, Unhappy, and Demotivated: The Impact of an Alone Mind-Set on Neurotic Individuals' Willpower. *Social Psychological and Personality Science* 7, no. 8 (2016): 818–827.

151 Daum, "Same Life, Higher Rent," *On Being 40(ish)*, ed. Lindsey Mead (New York: Simon & Schuster, 2019), 8.

152 Michael Cobb, *Single: Arguments for the Uncoupled* (New York: New York University Press, 2012), 21.

153 Rebecca K. Ratner and Rebecca W. Hamilton, "Inhibited from Bowling Alone," *Journal of Consumer Research* 42, no. 2 (2015): 266–283.

154 J. Victoria Sanders, *Single & Happy: The Party of Ones* (Los Gatos, CA: Smashwords, 2013).

155 Yuechen Wu, Rebecca W. Hamilton, Nicole You Jeung Kim, and Rebecca K. Ratner, "Navigating Shared Consumption Experiences: Clarity About a Partner's Interests Increases Enjoyment," *Journal of Marketing Research* 58, no. 3 (2021): 439–455.

156 Jess McHugh, "How to Eat Alone (and Like It)" *New York Times*, October 30, 2019, https://www.nytimes.com/2019/10/30/smarter-living/how-to-eat-alone-and-like-it.html.

157 Mary Madden and Lee Rainie, "Americans' Attitudes About Privacy, Security and Surveillance," Pew Research Center. May 20, 2015, https://www.pewresearch.org/internet/2015/05/20/americans-attitudes-about-privacy-security-and-surveillance/.

158 Donna Ward, *She I Dare Not Name: A Spinster's Meditations on Life* (Sydney: Allen & Unwin, 2021).

159 Bereznai, *Gay and Single . . . Forever?*, 129.

160 Anthony Storr, *Solitude: A Return to the Self* (New York: Ballantine Books, 1988).

161 Meals On Wheels, "Social Isolation Is as Deadly as Smoking Up to 15 Cigarettes a Day,"

advertisement, *New Yorker*, June 14, 2021, p. 5.

162 Robert J. Coplan, John M. Zelenski, and Julie C. Bowker, "Leave Well Enough Alone? The Costs and Benefits of Solitude," *Subjective Well-Being and Life Satisfaction*, ed. James E. Maddux (London: Routledge/Taylor & Francis, 2018), 129–147.

163 Ibid.

164 Maike Luhmann and Louise C. Hawkley, "Age Differences in Loneliness from Late Adolescence to Oldest Old Age," *Developmental Psychology* 52, no. 6 (2016): 943–959.

165 Robert J. Coplan, Will E. Hipson, and Julie C. Bowker, "Social Withdrawal and Aloneliness in Adolescence: Examining the Implications of Too Much and Not Enough Solitude," *Journal of Youth and Adolescence* 50, no. 6 (2021): 1219–1233.

166 Coplan et al., "Leave Well Enough Alone?" 129–147.

167 Helen Rosner, "Nigella Lawson Wants to Talk to People," *New Yorker*, April 14, 2021, https://www.newyorker.com/culture/the-new-yorker-interview/nigella-lawson-wants-to-talk-to-people.

168 Robert J. Coplan, Laura Ooi, and Will E. Hipson, "Solitary Activities from Early Childhood to Adolescence: Causes, Content, and Consequences," *The Handbook of Solitude: Psychological Perspectives on Social Isolatoin, Social Withdrawal, and Being Alone*, 2nd ed., eds. Robert J. Coplan, Julie C. Bowker, and Larry J. Nelson (New York: Wiley-Blackwell, 2021), 105–116.

169 Rufus, *Party of One*, 174.

170 Anna Machin, "Treasure Them," *Aeon*, June 4, 2021, https://aeon.co/essays/treasure-your-friends-the-top-of-your-love-hierarchy.

171 Peiqi Lu, Jeewon Oh, Katelin E. Leahy, and William J. Chopik, "Friendship Importance Around the World," *Frontiers in Psychology*, 11 (January 2021): Article 570839. https://doi.org/10.3389/fpsyg.2020.570839.

172 Bella DePaulo, "Single and Flourishing: Transcending the Deficit Narratives of Single Life," *Journal of Family Theory and Review* 15, no. 3 (2023): 398–411.

173 Roxane Gay, "Roxane Gay and Rebecca Traister Talk Sex, Female Friendship, and What It Means to Be Single Now," *Elle*, February 23, 2016, https://www.elle.com/life-love/sex-relationships/a34320/rebecca-traister-all-the-single-ladies-interview-roxane-gay/.

174 Naomi Gerstel, "Rethinking Families and Community: The Color, Class, and Centrality of Extended Kin Ties," *Sociological Forum* 26, no. 1 (2011): 1–20; Gerstel, Naomi, and Natalia Sarkisian, "Marriage: the Good, the Bad, and the Greedy," *Contexts*, 5, no. 4 (2006): 16-21; Sarkisian, Natalia, and Naomi Gerstel, "Does Singlehood Isolate or Integrate? Examining the Link Between Marital Status and Ties to Kin, Friends, and Neighbors," *Journal of Social and Personal Relationships 33, no. 3* (2016): 361–384.

175 Sarkisian and Gerstel, "Does Singlehood Isolate or Integrate?" 368.

176 Gerstel and Sarkisian, "Marriage," 16–21.

177 Robin Dunbar, *Friends: Understanding the Power of Our Most Important Relationships* (London: Little, Brown UK, 2022), 154.

178 Matthijs Kalmijn, "Shared Friendship Networks and the Life Course: An Analysis of Survey Data on Married and Cohabiting Couples," *Social Networks*, 25, no. 3 (2003): 231–249.

179 Kelly Musick and Larry Bumpass, "Reexamining the Case for Marriage: Union Formation and Changes in Well-Being," *Journal of Marriage and Family* 74, no. 1 (2012): 1–18.

180 Sonia Sotomayor, *My Beloved World* (New York: Vintage, 2014), 299.

181 Daniel Kahneman, Alan B. Krueger, David A. Schkade, Norbert Schwarz, and Arthur A. Stone, "A Survey Method for Characterizing Daily Life Experience: The Day Reconstruction Method," *Science* 306, no. 5702 (2004): 1776–1780.

182 Alexandra Fisher, Danu Anthony Stinson, Joanne V. Wood, John G. Holmes, and Jessica J. Cameron, "Singlehood and attunement of self-esteem to friendships," *Social Psychological and Personality Science* 12, no. 7 (2021): 1326–1334.

183 Kislev, "Social Capital, Happiness, and the Unmarried," 1475–1492.

184 Kislev, "How Do Relationship Desire and Sociability Relate to Each Other Among Singles?" 2634–2650.

185 Machin, "Treasure Them."

186 Sasha Roseneil, "Why We Should Care About Friends: An Argument for Queering the Care Imaginary in Social Policy," *Social Policy and Society* 3, no. 4 (2004): 409–419; Sasha Roseneil and Shelley Budgeon, "Cultures of Intimacy and Care Beyond 'the Family': Personal Life and Social Change in the

Early 21st Century," *Current Sociology* 52, no. 2 (2004): 135–159.

187 Roseneil, "Why We Should Care About Friends," 413.

188 Ibid.

189 Ibid.

190 Bereznai, *Gay and Single . . . Forever,* 163.

191 Briallen Hopper, *Hard to Love: Essays and Confessions* (London: Bloomsbury, 2019), 87.

192 Armistead Maupin, *Logical Family: A Memoir* (New York: Harper, 2017), 2.

193 Kath Weston, *Families We Choose: Lesbians, Gays, Kinship* (New York: Columbia University Press, 1991).

194 Bryant, "African American Fictive Kin."

195 Jessica D. Moorman, "Socializing Singlehood: Personal, Interpersonal, and Sociocultural Factors Shaping Black Women's Single Lives," *Psychology of Women Quarterly* 44, no. 4 (2020): 431–449.

196 Robert Joseph Taylor, Linda M. Chatters, Amanda Toler Woodward, and Edna Brown, "Racial and Ethnic Differences in Extended Family, Friendship, Fictive Kin, and Congregational Informal Support Networks," *Family Relations* 62, no. 4 (2013): 609–624.

197 E. Kay Trimberger, *The New Single Woman* (Boston, MA: Beacon Press, 2005), 249.

198 Miko Lee and Jalena Keane-Lee, hosts, "Sex Positivity," Apex Express (podcast), December 2, 2021, https://kpfa.org/episode/apex-express-december-2-2021/.

199 Heather F. Fuller, Kristine J. Ajrouch, and Toni C. Antonucci, "The Convoy Model and Later-Life Family Relationships," *Journal of Family Theory and Review* 12, no. 2 (2020): 126–146.

200 TallBear, "Making Love and Relations."

201 Vivek H. Murthy, *Together: The Healing Power of Human Connection in a Sometimes Lonely World* (New York: Harper Wave, 2020), 5.

202 Elaine O. Cheung, Wendi L. Gardner, and Jason F. Anderson, "Emotionships: Examining People's Emotion-Regulation Relationships and Their Consequences for Well-Being," *Social Psychological and Personality Science* 6, no. 4 (2015): 407–414.

203 Bella DePaulo, "How Many Americans Want to Be Single? Results of 5 Studies." *Psychology Today*, September 20, 2017, https://www.psychologytoday.com/intl/blog/living-single/201709/how-many-americans-want-be-single-results-5-studies.

204 Cathy Goodwin, "How Hospitals Do Us Wrong," *Psychology Today*, March 26, 2016, https://www.psychologytoday.com/intl/blog/living-single/201603/how-hospitals-do-us-wrong.

205 Whoopi Goldberg, *If Someone Says "You Complete Me," RUN!: Whoopi's Big Book of Relationships* (New York: Hachette Books, 2015), 156.

206 Rhaina Cohen, "What If Friendship, Not Marriage, Was at the Center of Life?" *The Atlantic*, October 20, 2020, https://www.theatlantic.com/family/archive/2020/10/people-who-prioritize-friendship-over-romance/616779/.

207 Ibid.

208 Machin, "Treasure Them."

209 Olga Stavrova and Dongning Ren, "Is More Always Better? Examining the Nonlinear Association of Social Contact Frequency with Physical Health and Longevity," *Social Psychological and Personality Science* 12, no. 6 (2021): 1058–1070.

210 Ibid.

211 Ibid.

212 Carol S. Kahn, "Not the Loneliest Number: A Grounded Theory Study of Never-Married Single Adults and Attachment," Unpublished doctoral dissertation, Drexel University, 2011.

213 Keturah Kendrick, *No Thanks: Black, Female, and Living in the Martyr-Free Zone* (Berkeley, CA: She Writes Press, 2019), 43.

214 National Health Service, "Female Sterilisation: Your Contraception Guide," accessed January 20, 2023, https://www.nhs.uk/conditions/contraception/female-sterilisation/.

215 Olga Khazan, "How People Decide Whether to Have Children," *The Atlantic*, May 22, 2107, https://www.theatlantic.com/health/archive/2017/05/how-people-decide-whether-to-have-children/527520/.

216 James Gallagher, "Fertility Rate: 'Jaw-Dropping' Global Crash in Children Being Born," BBC, July 15, 2020, https://www.bbc.com/news/health-53409521.

217 Tayelor Valerio, Brian Knop, Rose M. Kreider, and Wan He, "Childless Older Americans: 2018," US Census Bureau, Current Population Reports (Washington, DC: US Government Printing Office, August 2021), 70–173.

218 Anna Brown, "Growing Share of Childless Adults in US Don't Expect to Ever Have Children," Pew Research Center, November 19, 2021, https://www.pewresearch.org/fact-tank/2021/11/19/growing-share-of-childless-adults-in-u-s-dont-expect-to-ever-have-children/.

219 Karen Benjamin Guzzo, "Childbearing Desires, Intentions, and Attitudes Among Women 40–44," *Family Profiles* No. 9, (Bowling Green, OH: National Center for Family & Marriage Research, 2018). https://www.bgsu.edu/ncfmr/resources/data/family-profiles/guzzo-childbearing-desires-intent-attitudes-women-40-44-fp-18-09.html.

220 DePaulo and Morris, "Singles in Society and in Science," 57–83.

221 Kiley Hurst, "Rising Share of Americans See Women Raising Children on Their Own, Cohabitation as Bad for Society," Pew Research Center, March 11, 2022, https://www.pewresearch.org/fact-tank/2022/03/11/rising-share-of-americans-see-women-raising-children-on-their-own-cohabitation-as-bad-for-society/.

222 Jennifer Watling Neal and Zachary P. Neal, "Prevalence and Characteristics of Childfree Adults in Michigan (USA)," *PLOS ONE* 16, no. 6 (2021): e0252528.

223 Amy V. Andrada, "Scarlet Letter Effect: Evidence of a Single Mother Narrative," Doctoral Dissertation, University of Edinburgh, 2022, https://era.ed.ac.uk/handle/1842/39097.

224 Crisell, "The Rise of the Alpha Single," 26.

225 Joseph Chamie, "Out-of-Wedlock Births Rise Worldwide," YaleGlobal Online, March 16, 2017, https://archive-yaleglobal.yale.edu/content/out-wedlock-births-rise-worldwide.

226 Amanda Barroso, "With a Potential 'Baby Bust' on the Horizon, Key Facts about Fertility in the US Before the Pandemic," Pew Research Center. May 7, 2021, https://www.pewresearch.org/fact-tank/2021/05/07/with-a-potential-baby-bust-on-the-horizon-key-facts-about-fertility-in-the-u-s-before-the-pandemic/.

227 Brown, "Growing Share of Childless Adults in US Don't Expect to Ever Have Children."

228 Ibid.

229 Spielmann et al., "Settling for Less Out of Fear of Being Single."

230 DePaulo, *Singled Out*, 169–184.

231 Simon Chapple, "Child Well-Being and Sole-Parent Family Structure in the OECD," *OECD Social, Employment and Migration Working Papers*, no. 82, OECD Publishing, 2009, https://www.oecd-ilibrary.org/social-issues-migration-health/child-well-being-and-sole-parent-family-structure-in-the-oecd_225407362040.

232 Shannon Cavanagh, "An Analysis of New Census Data on Family Structure, Education, and Income," Council on Contemporary Families, February 26, 2015, https://sites.utexas.edu/contemporaryfamilies/2015/02/26/family-structure-education-income/; Matthew T. Usevitch and Mikaela J. Dufur, "When Single Parents Marry: Do Children Benefit Academically?" *Family Relations* 70, no. 4 (2021): 1206–1221.

233 Suet-ling Pong, Jaap Dronkers, and Gillian Hampden-Thompson, "Family Policies and Children's School Achievement in Single- Versus Two-Parent Families," *Journal of Marriage and Family* 65, no. 3 (2003): 681-699.

234 Sumi Rabindrakumar, "Family Portrait: Single Parent Families and Transitions Over Time," University of Sheffield, June 1, 2018, https://www.basw.co.uk/system/files/resources/Sheffield_Solutions_Modern_Families.pdf.

235 Rena L. Repetti, Shelley E. Taylor, and Teresa E. Seaman, "Risky Families: Family Social Environments and the Mental and Physical Health of Offspring," *Psychological Bulletin* 128, no. 2 (2002): 330–366.

236 Susan Golombok, Sophie Zadeh, Susan Imrie, Vanessa Smith, and Tabitha Freeman, "Single Mothers by Choice: Mother-Child Relationships and Children's Psychological Adjustment," *Journal of Family Psychology* 30, no. 4 (2016): 409–418.

237 Lyz Lenz, "The Subversive Joy of Being a Single Mother," Substack, June 8, 2022, https://lyz.substack.com/p/the-subversive-joy-of-being-a-single?s=w.

238 American Psychological Association, "Single Parenting and Today's Family," October 31, 2019, https://www.apa.org/topics/parenting/single-parent.

239 Joanna R. Pepin, Liana C. Sayer, and Lynne M. Casper, "'Marital Status and Mothers' Time Use: Childcare, Housework, Leisure, and Sleep," *Demography* 55, no. 1 (2018): 107–133.

240 Lara Bazelon, "All the Single Mothers," *Slate*, May 11, 2019, https://slate.com/human-interest/2019/05/single-moms-fewer-chores-free-time-married.html.

241 Ibid.

242 Dani McClain, *We Live for the We: The Political Power of Black Motherhood* (New York, NY: Bold Type Books, 2019), 61.

243 Ibid.

244 Thomas DeLeire and Ariel Kalil, "Good Things Come in Threes: Single-Parent Multigenerational Family Structures and Adolescent Adjustment," *Demography* 39, no. 2 (2002): 393–413.

245 April (blogger), "I'm a Homeowner!!" *It's All About Balance* (blog), December 23, 2019. http://www.singleparentbalance.org/2019/.

246 Lenz, "The Subversive Joy of Being a Single Mother."

247 Matt Peiken, "Survival in the DNA of Malaprop's Bookstore and its Singularly Focused Founder," Blue Ridge Public Radio, February 6, 2019, https://www.bpr.org/arts-performance/2019-02-06/survival-in-the-dna-of-malaprops-bookstore-and-its-singularly-focused-founder#stream/0.

248 Ibid.

249 Amy Blackstone, *Childfree by Choice: The Movement Redefining Family and Creating a New Age of Independence* (New York: Dutton, 2019), 127.

250 Dani McClain, *We Live for the We: The Political Power of Black Motherhood* (New York, NY: Bold Type Books, 2019), 62.

251 Pamela Haag, "The UnQueered World: Take a Walk on the Mild Side," Big Think, January 26, 2013, https://bigthink.com/articles/the-unqueered-world-take-a-walk-on-the-mild-side/.

252 Kislev, "The Sexual Activity and Sexual Satisfaction of Singles in the Second Demographic Transition," 726–738.

253 Amy Gahran, *Stepping Off the Escalator: Uncommon Love and Life* (Boulder, CO: Off the Escalator Enterprises, 2017).

254 Haili Blassingame, "My Choice Isn't Marriage or Loneliness," *New York Times*, April 4, 2021.

255 Angela Chen, *Ace: What Asexuality Reveals About Desire, Society, and the Meaning of Sex* (Boston, MA: Beacon Press, 2021), 3–4.

256 Ibid.

257 Asexuals.net (@AsexualsNet), "Think of someone you aren't attached to. Now imagine that is how you feel about everyone. The end," Twitter, April 23, 2022, 11:46 a.m. https://twitter.com/AsexualsNet/status/1517937948766973954.

258 Michael Gold, "The ABCs of L. G. B. T. Q. I. A. +" *New York Times*, June 21, 2018. https://www.nytimes.com/2018/06/21/style/lgbtq-gender-language.html.

259 Chen, *Ace*.

260 Kislev, "The Sexual Activity and Sexual Satisfaction of Singles in the Second Demographic Transition," 726–738.

261 Jean M. Twenge, Ryne A. Sherman, and Brooke E. Wells, "Declines in Sexual Frequency among American Adults, 1989–2014," *Archives of Sexual Behavior* 46 (March 2017): 2389–2401.

262 Kate Julian, "Why Are Young People Having So Little Sex?" *The Atlantic*, December 2018. https://www.theatlantic.com/magazine/archive/2013/12/the-sex-recession/573949/.

263 Buchanan, Kyle, "Linda Hamilton Fled Hollywood, but 'Terminator' Still Found Her," *New York Times*, updated November 4, 2019, https://www.nytimes.com/2019/09/03/movies/linda-hamilton-terminator.html.

264 Ed Anderson, "Sex Is Overrated." Uncoupled, May 1, 2022, https://un-coupled.com/?p=217.

265 Lucas Bradley, "I've Never Had Sexual Relations. I'm No 'Virgin,'" Medium, February 12, 2022, https://medium.com/@lucasbradley/ive-never-had-sexual-relations-i-m-no-virgin-46f6445b9ec.

266 Ibid.

267 Johnson, *At the Center of All Beauty*, 193.

268 Twenge et al., "Declines in Sexual Frequency among American Adults, 1989–2014."

269 Kelsey Borresen, "What It Means to Be 'Aromantic,' According to Aromantic People," HuffPost, June 3, 2022, https://www.huffpost.com/entry/what-does-it-mean-to-be-aromantic_n_5bb501cee4b01470d04de20d.

270 Ibid.

271 Xenia Taliotis, "I'm a Relationship Virgin: I'm 54 and Have Never Had a Boyfriend," *Guardian*, October 28, 2017, https://www.theguardian.com/lifeandstyle/2017/oct/28/relationship-virgin-never-boyfriend-single.

272 Sana Panjwani, "I'm 27, I've Never Been in a Relationship, & I'm Starting to Think I Never Will Be," *Refinery29*, September 13, 2021, https://www.refinery29.com/en-us/2021/09/10648252/happy-single-never-had-a-relationship.

273 Ibid.

274 DePaulo and Morris, "Singles in Society and in Science," 57–83.

275 Mollie Quirk, "I've Never Had Sex, a Boyfriend, or Even My First Kiss—and I'm Not Sure I Ever Will. Here's Why I'm Totally

Fine with That," *Glamour*, February 14, 2022. https://www.glamourmagazine.co.uk/article/single-virgin-valentines-day.

276 Brooke Douglas and Pamela Orpinas, "Social Misfit or Normal Development? Students Who Do Not Date," *Journal of School Health* 89, no. 10 (2019): 783–790.

277 Kara Joyner and J. Richard Udry, "You Don't Bring Me Anything But Down: Adolescent Romance and Depression," *Journal of Health and Social Behavior* 41, no. 4 (2000): 369–391.

278 Ibid.

279 Matthew D. Johnson, Franz J. Neyer, and Christine Finn, "Subjective Well-Being Across Partnerships," *Journal of Family Psychology* 35, no. 4 (2021): 546–551.

280 Luhmann et al., "Subjective Well-Being and Adaptation to Life Events," 592–615.

281 Douglas and Orpinas, "Social Misfit or Normal Development?" 783–790.

282 Jonathon J. Beckmeyer and Shannon Cromwell, "Romantic Relationship Status and Emerging Adult Well-Being: Accounting for Romantic Relationship Interest," *Emerging Adulthood* 7, no. 4 (2019): 304–308.

283 Glenn I. Roisman, Ann S. Masten, J. Douglas Coatsworth, and Auke Tellegen, "Salient and Emerging Developmental Tasks in the Transition to Adulthood," *Child Development* 75, no. 1 (2004): 123–133.

284 Catherine Clifford, "On Running and Asexual Embodiment," *Aze*, June 15, 2019, https://azejournal.com/article/2019/6/3/on-running-and-asexual-embodiment.

285 Dunbar, *Friends*, 156.

286 Alix Strauss, "Losing at Love? A Coach May Help You Win," *New York Times*, March 17, 2022, section D, p. 4.

287 Tippett, "Sandra Cisneros."

288 Barbara Hillary, "Barbara Hillary, Commencement Speaker 2017, The New School," YouTube video. May 23, 2017.

289 Katharine Q. Seelye, "Barbara Hillary, 88, Trailblazer on Top (and Bottom) of the World, Dies," *New York Times*, November 26, 2019, https://www.nytimes.com/2019/11/26/us/barbara-hillary-dead.html.

290 Lauren Collins, "The Latest Dreams of Barbara Hillary, the First African-American Woman to Travel to the North Pole," *New Yorker*, July 26, 2019, https://www.newyorker.com/culture/culture-desk/the-latest-dreams-of-barbara-hillary-the-first-african-american-woman-to-travel-to-the-north-pole.

291 Ibid.

292 Ibid.

293 Seelye, "Barbara Hillary, 88, Trailblazer on Top (and Bottom) of the World, Dies."

294 Hillary, "Barbara Hillary, Commencement Speaker 2017, The New School."

295 Lauren Collins, "True North," *New Yorker*, March 26, 2007, https://www.newyorker.com/magazine/2007/03/26/true-north-4.

296 Collins, "The Latest Dreams of Barbara Hillary."

297 Kendrick, *No Thanks*, 25.

298 Anna Brown, "Nearly Half of US Adults Say Dating Has Gotten Harder for Most People in the Last 10 Years," Pew Research Center. August 20, 2020, https://www.pewresearch.org/social-trends/2020/08/20/nearly-half-of-u-s-adults-say-dating-has-gotten-harder-for-most-people-in-the-last-10-years/.

299 Ibid.

300 Ibid.

301 Anne Böger and Oliver Huxhold, "The Changing Relationship Between Partnership Status and Loneliness: Effects Related to Aging and Historical Time," *The Journals of Gerontology: Series B: Psychological Sciences and Social Sciences* 75, no. 7 (2020): 1423–1432; Park, Yoobin, Elizabeth Page-Gould, and Geoff MacDonald, "Satisfying Singlehood as a Function of Age and Cohort: Satisfaction with Being Single Increases with Age After Midlife," *Psychology and Aging* 37, no. 5 (2022): 626–636.

302 Brown, "Nearly Half of US Adults Say Dating Has Gotten Harder for Most People in the Last 10 Years."

303 Park et al., "Satisfying Singlehood as a Function of Age and Cohort," 626–636.

304 Brown, "Nearly Half of US Adults Say Dating Has Gotten Harder for Most People in the Last 10 Years."

305 Jane Gross, "Why Some of Us Reject Marriage," *Next Avenue*, February 21, 2013. https://www.nextavenue.org/why-some-us-reject-marriage/.

306 Ibid.

307 Brown, "Nearly Half of US Adults Say Dating Has Gotten Harder for Most People in the Last 10 Years."

308 Böger and Huxhold, "The Changing Relationship Between Partnership Status and Loneliness."

309 Park et al., "Satisfying Singlehood as a Function of Age and Cohort," 626–636.

310 Marks and Lambert, "Marital Status Continuity and Change Among Young and Midlife Adults," 652–686.

311 Park et al., "Satisfying Singlehood as a Function of Age and Cohort," 633.

312 Marks and Lambert, "Marital Status Continuity and Change Among Young and Midlife Adults," 652–686.

313 Maria Eisman, Kene Henkens, and Matthijs Kalmijn, "Why Singles Prefer to Retire Later," *Research on Aging* 4, no. 10 (2019): 936–960.

314 Julie Cwikel, Helen Gramotnev, and Christina Lee, "Never-married childless women in Australia: Health and social circumstances in older age," *Social Science & Medicine* 62, no. 8 (2006) 1991–2001.

315 Tetyana Pudrovska, Scott Schieman, and Deborah Carr, "Strains of Singlehood in Later Life: Do Race and Gender Matter?" *The Journals of Gerontology: Series B* 61, no. 6 (2006): S315–S322.

316 Yoobin Park, Elizabeth Page-Gould, and Geoff MacDonald, "Satisfying Singlehood as a Function of Age and Cohort: Satisfaction with Being Single Increases with Age After Midlife." *Psychology and Aging* 37, no. 5 (2022): 626–636.

317 Colette Thayer, "Solo Agers Are Optimistic About Quality of Life," AARP Research, February 2021, https://www.aarp.org/research/topics/life/info-2021/solo-agers-attitudes-experiences.html.

318 Kislev, *Happy Singlehood*, 93.

319 Jan Eckhard, "Social Isolation as a Consequence of Transitions in Partner Relationships: How Formations and Endings of Partner Relationships Affect the Risk of Disconnectedness," *Journal of Family Research* 33, no. 1 (2021), 48.

320 Ibid.

321 Bronnie Ware, *Top Five Regrets of the Dying: A Life Transformed by the Dearly Departing* (Carlsbad, CA: Hay House, 2019), 135.

322 Lu et al., "Friendship Importance Around the World."

323 Matthew R. Wright and Susan L. Brown, "Psychological Well-Being Among Older Adults: The Role of Partnership Status," *Journal of Marriage and Family* 79, no. 3 (2017): 833–849.

324 Ashley E. Ermer and Christine M. Proulx, "Associations Between Social Connectedness, Emotional Well-Being, and Self-Rated Health Among Older Adults: Differences by Relationship Status," *Research on Aging* 41, no. 4 (2019): 336–361.

325 Brandy Renee McCann and Katherine R. Allen, "Romantic Forecasts in Later Life: Older Single Women's Perspectives on Family and Kin Relationships," *Journal of Family Issues* 39, no. 3 (2018): 747–770.

326 Ibid.

327 Erin S. Lavender-Stott and Katherine R. Allen, "Not Alone: Family Experiences Across the Life Course of Single, Baby Boom Sexual-Minority Women," *Family Relations* 72, no. 1 (2023): 140–158.

328 Voorpostel, Marieke. "Just Like Family: Fictive Kin Relationships in the Netherlands." *The Journals of Gerontology: Series B* 68, no. 5 (2013): 816-824.

329 Thayer, "Solo Agers Are Optimistic About Quality of Life."

330 Paul Taylor, Rich Morin, Kim Parker, D'Vera Cohn, and Wendy Wang, "Growing Old in America: Expectations vs. Reality," Pew Research Center, June 29, 2009, https://www.pewresearch.org/social-trends/2009/06/29/growing-old-in-america-expectations-vs-reality/.

331 Jennifer C. Lay, Theresa Pauly, Peter Graf, Atiya Mahmood, and Christine A. Hoppmann, "Choosing Solitude: Age Differences in Situational and Affective Correlates of Solitude-Seeking in Midlife and Older Adulthood," *Journals of Gerontology B: Psychological Sciences* 75, no. 3 (2020): 483–493.

332 Netta Weinstein, Thuy-vy Nguyen, and Heather Hansen, "What Time Alone Offers: Narratives of Solitude from Adolescence to Older Adulthood," *Frontiers in Psychology* 12 (2021): Article 714518.

333 G. Clare Wenger and Vanessa Burholt, "Changes in Levels of Social Isolation and Loneliness Among Older People in a Rural Area: A Twenty-Year Longitudinal Study," *Canadian Journal on Aging* 23, no. 2 (2004): 115–127.

334 Thayer, "Solo Agers Are Optimistic About Quality of Life."

335 Melanie D. Sereny and Danan Gu, "Living Arrangement Concordance and Its Association with Self-Rated Health Among Institutionalized and Community-Residing Older Adults in China," *Journal of Cross-Cultural Gerontology* 26, no. 3 (2011): 239–259.

336 Sarah Lamb, *Being Single in India: Stories of Gender, Exclusion, and Possibility* (Oakland, CA: University of California Press, 2022), 91.

337 Taylor et al., "Growing Old in America."

338 DelFattore, "Death by Stereotype," 982.

339 Amelia Karraker and Kenzie Latham, "In Sickness and in Health? Physical Illness as a Risk Factor for Marital Dissolution in Later Life," *Journal of Health and Social Behavior* 56, no. 3 (2015): 420–35.

340 Jay Teachman, "Work-Related Health Limitations, Education, and the Risk of Marital Disruption," *Journal of Marriage and Family* 72, no. 4 (2010): 919–932.

341 Niall Bolger, Mark Foster, Amiram D. Vinokur, and Rosanna Ng, "Close Relationships and Adjustment to a Life Crisis: The Case of Breast Cancer," *Journal of Personality and Social Psychology* 70, no. 2 (1996): 283–294.

342 Candyce Kroenke, Laura D. Kubzansky, Eva S. Schernhammer, Michelle D. Holmes, and Ichiro Kawachi, "Social Networks, Social Support, and Survival After Breast Cancer Diagnosis," *Journal of Clinical Oncology* 24, no. 7 (2006): 1105–1110.

343 Liz Spencer and Ray Pahl, *Rethinking Friendship: Hidden Solidarities Today* (Princeton, NJ: Princeton University Press, 2006).

344 Kristina Scharp, "What Is Family Estrangement? A Relationship Expert Describes the Problem and Research Agenda," *The Conversation*, October 14, 2021, https://theconversation.com/what-is-family-estrangement-a-relationship-expert-describes-the-problem-and-research-agenda-164852.

345 Kim Parker and Juliana Menasce Horowitz, "Family Support in Graying Societies: How Americans, Germans and Italians Are Coping with an Aging Population," Pew Research Center, May 21, 2015.

346 Jung-Hwa Ha and Deborah Carr, "The Effect of Parent-Child Geographic Proximity on Widowed Parents' Psychological Adjustment and Social Integration," *Research on Aging* 27, no. 5 (2005): 578–610.

347 Jagriti Gangopadhyay, "Examining the Lived Experiences of Ageing Among Older Adults Living Alone in India," *Ageing Issues and Responses in India*, ed. Mala Kapur Shankardass (Singapore: Springer, Singapore, 2020) 207–219.

348 Ketaki Chowkhani, "Successfully Aging Alone: Long-Term Singlehood and Care during COVID-19 in India," *Eldercare issues in China and India*, eds. Longtao He and Jagriti Gangopadhyay (London: Routledge, 2022), 145–154.

349 Barbara Ellen, "Loneliness Is One Thing. A Happy Loner Quite Another," *Guardian*, June 21, 2014, https://www.theguardian.com/commentisfree/2014/jun/22/britain-loneliness-capital-isolation-being-alone?CMP=fb_gu.

350 Glenys Caswell, *Dying Alone: Challenging Assumptions* (Cham, Switzerland: Palgrave Macmillan, 2022).

351 Ann Neumann, "Death Trips: Accessorizing the Final Exit Lane," *The Baffler*, no. 35, June 2017, https://thebaffler.com/salvos/death-trips-neumann.

352 Bella DePaulo, Think Again, "A Contrarian's View of Dying Alone: Guest Post by 'Think Again,'" *Psych Central*, September 18, 2016, https://psychcentral.com/blog/single-at-heart/2016/09/a-contrarians-view-of-dying-alone-guest-post-by-think-again.

353 Ruth Wilson, "The Painful Decisions I Made After 50 Years of Marriage," *The Sydney Morning Herald*, March 27, 2022, https://www.smh.com.au/lifestyle/life-and-relationships/the-painful-decisions-i-made-after-50-years-of-marriage-20220323-p5a75i.html.

354 Ibid.

355 Raley and Sweeney, "Divorce, Repartnering, and Stepfamilies: A Decade in Review," 81–99.

356 Susan L. Brown, I-Fen Lin, Anna M. Hammersmith, and Matthew R. Wright, "Repartnering Following Gray Divorce: The Roles of Resources and Constraints for Women and Men," *Demography* 56, no. 2 (2019): 503–523.

357 Renee Stepler, "Led by Baby Boomers, Divorce Rates Climb for America's 50+ Population," Pew Research Center, March 9, 20.

358 Renee Stepler, "Led by Baby Boomers, Divorce Rates Climb for America's 50+ Population," Pew Research Center, March 9, 2017, https://www.pewresearch.org/fact-tank/2017/03/09/led-by-baby-boomers-divorce-rates-climb-for-americas-50-population/.

359 Deirdre Bair, "The 40-Year Itch," *New York Times*, June 3, 2010. https://www.nytimes.com/2010/06/04/opinion/04bair.html.

360 Ibid.

361 Ware, *The Top Five Regrets of the Dying*, 37.

362 DePaulo and Morris, "Singles in Society, and in Science," 57–83.

363 Ibid.

364 Ibid.

365 Luhmann et al., "Subjective Well-Being and Adaptation to Life Events," 592–615.

366 I have repeatedly critiqued that claim, and others like it; for example, in *Marriage vs. Single Life: How Science and the Media Got It So Wrong* (Self-published: CreateSpace, 2015), *Singled Out: How Singles Are Stereotyped, Stigmatized, and Ignored, and Still Live Happily Ever After* (New York: St. Martin's Griffin, 2006), and "Get Married, Get Healthy? Maybe Not." *New York Times*, May 25, 2017, https://www.nytimes.com/2017/05/25/opinion/marriage-health-study.html?ref=opinion.

367 Wendy L. Morris and Brittany K. Osburn, "Do You Take This Marriage? Perceived Choice over Marital Status Affects the Stereotypes of Single and Married People," *Singlehood from Individual and Social Perspectives*, ed. Katarzyna Adamczyk (Krakow, Poland: Libron, 2016), 145–162.

368 Gal Slonim, Nurit Gur-Yaish, and Ruth Katz, "By Choice or Circumstance?: Stereotypes of and Feelings about Single People," *Studia Psychologica* 57 no. 1 (2015): 35–47.

369 DePaulo, *Singled Out*, 4.

370 Marsh, *The Love Jones Cohort*, 69, 72.

371 Nancy Leong, "Negative Identity," *Southern California Law Review* 88, no. 5 (2015): 1395.

372 Martin V. Day, Aaron C. Kay, John G. Holmes, and Jaime L. Napier, "System Justification and the Defense of Committed Relationship Ideology," *Journal of Personality and Social Psychology* 101, no. 2 (2011): 291–306.

373 Bella DePaulo, "Single and Flourishing: Transcending the Deficit Narratives of Single Life," *Journal of Family Theory and Review*, Volume 15, Issue 3: 389–411; Bella DePaulo, "Toward a Positive Psychology of Single Life." *Positive Psychology: Established and emerging issues*, edited by Dana Dunn (New York: Routledge, 2018), 251–275

374 Andrew J. Cherlin, "Degrees of Change: An Assessment of the Deinstitutionalization of Marriage Thesis," *Journal of Marriage and Family* 82, no. 1 (2020): 62–80.

375 US Census Bureau, Table MS-2, "Estimated Median Age at First Marriage, by Sex: 1890 to the Present."

376 Kim Parker and Wendy Wang, "Record Share of Americans Have Never Married," Pew Research Center, September 24, 2014. https://www.pewresearch.org/social-trends/2014/09/24/record-share-of-americans-have-never-married/.

377 Pamela J. Smock, Wendy D. Manning, and Meredith Porter, "'Everything's There Except Money': How Money Shapes Decisions to Marry Among Cohabitors," *Journal of Marriage and Family* 67, no. 3 (2005): 680–696.

378 Kim Parker and Renee Stepler, "As US Marriage Rate Hovers at 50%, Education Gap in Marital Status Widens." Pew Research Center, September 14, 2017, https://www.pewresearch.org/short-reads/2017/09/14/as-u-s-marriage-rate-hovers-at-50-education-gap-in-marital-status-widens/.

379 US Government Accountability Office, *Defense of Marriage Act: Update to Prior Report*, 2004, https://www.gao.gov/products/gao-04-353r; DePaulo, *Singlism: What It Is, Why It Matters, and How to Stop It* (Charleston, SC: DoubleDoor Books, 2011).

380 DePaulo, *Singlism*.

381 Jaclyn Geller, *Moving Past Marriage: Why We Should Ditch Marital Privilege, Eschew Relationship-Status Discrimination, and Embrace Non-Marital History* (Jersey City, NJ: Cleis Press, 2023).

382 Naomi Cahn, "Reflections on Singlehood," *Washington University Journal of Law and Policy* 72, no. 1 (2023): 27–50.

383 US Equal Employment Opportunity Commission, *Prohibited Employment Policies/Practices*, accessed May 19, 2023, https://www.eeoc.gov/prohibited-employment-policiespractices.

384 Angelica Malin, "I Got More Respect for Marrying Than for My Career," *Grazia*, February 2023, 53.

385 Wendy L. Morris, Stacey Sinclair, and Bella M. DePaulo, "No Shelter for Singles: The Perceived Legitimacy of Marital Status Discrimination," *Group Processes & Intergroup Relations* 10, no. 4 (2007): 457–470.

386 In "Uncoupling," law professors Naomi Cahn and June Carbone argue that for all Americans to have security and stability, benefits and protections should be uncoupled from marriage and employment.

387 Vicki Larson, "Parents, Stop Agonizing Over Your Millennial Kid's Love Life," *OMG Chronicles*, July 23, 2019, http://omgchronicles.vickilarson.com/2019/07/23/parents-millennial-sex-love-dating/.

388 Razi Shachar, Tali Leshem, Jamina Rosenberg, Aya Schmidt, and Vivy Schmuely, "Ex-

ploring Discourses That Affect Therapists Regarding Single Women," *Journal of Feminist Family Therapy* 25, no. 4 (2013), 272.

389 Ibid, 275.

390 McClain, *We Live for the We*.

391 Joan DelFattore, "Death by Stereotype? Cancer Treatment in Unmarried Patients," *The New England Journal of Medicine* 381, no 10 (2019): 982.

392 Ibid, 983.

393 Storr, *Solitude*, 29.

394 Sharon Ost-Mor, Yuval Palgi, and Dikla Segel-Karpas, "Exploring Gaps in Positive Solitude Perceptions: Older Adults vs. Gerontology Professionals," *International Psychogeriatrics* 33, no. 12 (2021), 1253–1263.

395 Bella DePaulo, *How We Live Now: Redefining Home and Family in the 21st Century* (New York: Atria Books, 2015).

396 Sasha Roseneil, "It's Time to End the Tyranny of Coupledom," *Guardian*, November 14, 2020, https://www.theguardian.com/commentisfree/2020/nov/14/coupledom-couple-norm-social-change.

397 Catherine Powell, "Up from Marriage: Freedom, Solitude, and Individual Autonomy in the Shadow of Marriage Equality," *Fordham Law Review* 84 no. 1 (2015): 74–75.

Acknowledgments

Thank you to the forty-one people who generously shared their life stories with me. You are the heart and soul of this book. Thanks, too, to the hundreds of others who have told me about aspects of their lives over the years, especially those who graciously agreed to have their stories recounted in *Single at Heart*. My heart has been warmed by the untold numbers of strangers who have let me know that they too are single at heart. I am also indebted to the people from around the world—now numbering more than twenty thousand—who answered the online *Single at Heart* quiz.

I dedicated my first book about single life, *Singled Out*, "to Susan Hurt, an extraordinary friend." All these years later, she is even more extraordinary. I am so fortunate to have had her in my life for decades. Thanks, too, to Rebecca Zwick, Alicia Rosenthal, Nancy Collins, Bobbie Spellman, Karen Taylor, and Per Wehn, the kinds of friends everyone should be so fortunate to have.

Thanks to Kris Marsh, not just for her groundbreaking work on adults who are single and living alone in the black middle class, but also for her sparkling company over seaside lunches.

Thanks to the inspiring scholar, educator, and friend, Amy Andrada. She does important work on single mothers and she knows how to share her ideas engagingly.

Thanks to Wendy Morris, who collaborated with me on my earliest studies of single people and whose insights have stayed with me to this day. Weylin Sternglanz and I collaborated too; our research was not about single people, but his years of expressing interest in that work make me happy.

Thanks to the group of single women I met through NextDoor, who came together for lunch every Friday during the summer when I was trying to find a home for *Single at Heart* and who were wonderfully supportive.

Thanks to Julia Ortega, Luis Ortega, and Teresa Curiel for many years of warmth and kindness.

I am indebted to the many coupled people who have been my allies and my friends throughout my life. They really get what single at heart means, and what it means to me.

Many of the people for whom I feel affection and gratitude are people I've never met in person. Joan DelFattore is one of my favorites. I trust her judgment about matters of the single at heart, perhaps more than anyone else's. She is also doing great things for all single people with her research on issues in the treatment of single people by the medical community.

I've never met Ketaki Chowkhani either—we live nine thousand miles apart—but I am completely taken by her brilliance, her heart, her many talents, and all she is doing to put the study of single people on the map. She is the number one reason I am optimistic about the future of singlehood studies.

Jackie Geller has been in the fray for decades, arguing compellingly for fairness for people who are not married. Elyakim Kislev has brought a vibrancy to the study of single life with his impressive and wide-ranging research spanning dozens of nations. Naomi Cahn played a more pivotal role in making this book happen than I could ever have imagined. She is also helping many other scholars of single life with her efforts and creativity in bringing us together. Krysten M. Fikes has treated me to many nuggets of insight and wisdom. Craig Wynne is another point of hope for the future of singlehood studies.

Single at Heart is a better book because of all the people who provided feedback along the way. I signed up to consult with Jane Friedman before I wrote a proposal, and in return I received not just great advice, but kindness and encouragement too. Susan Hurt, Joan DelFattore, and Rebecca Zwick were there for me during the trying times of proposal-writing and heartbreaking rejections. Jackie Geller, Joan DelFattore, and Amy Andrada gifted me with their close reading of early drafts of the book. Whole communities of people helped. In 2015 I started the Facebook group the Community of Single People and its members have been a source of inspiration and wisdom ever since. I shared early drafts of the advice sections of my chapters with them, as well as the section on the principles and values of the single at heart, and those sections were much improved by their feedback. I'm also indebted to the members of two other newer Facebook groups, Fairness for Single People and Single People at Heart, who were also sources of insights and enthusiasm.

The feedback I got repeatedly on my earlier drafts of *Single at Heart* was to add more of my own personal stories. I did that, though a bit reluctantly. I think that in some ways, other single people are better examples of what it means to be single at heart than I am. And I'm acutely aware of some of my coupled friends and relatives who have some single at heart kinds of strengths that surpass my own. I admire them all.

You, dear readers, are welcome to mock me for this one, but I am grateful for Twitter, especially when it was still called Twitter. It has been a fun place to meet new people and greet the old, savor their bite-sized morsels of smarts and snark, and learn about new research, sometimes even before it is published.

My deepest gratitude goes to my agent, Bridget Matzie. I had heard amazing things about her before we connected, but they were all wrong—she's even better than that! I never knew that an agent could be so dedicated to a project. I will be forever grateful. Thanks to Erin Files and Mags Chmielarczyk, also of Aevitas Creative, who got *Single at Heart* into the hands and hearts of readers beyond the English-speaking world— very exciting!

Many thanks to the whole crew at Apollo Publishers: publisher and director of editorial Julia Abramoff; publisher and director of sales Alex Merrill; associate editor Drew Anderla; designer Maeve Norton; and publicist ErinNicole Conti. They made my *Single at Heart* dreams come true.

As I write this, I have just started working with the publicist Leah Paulos, founder of The Press Shop, but I am already impressed and grateful.

I am thankful for my beloved siblings, Peter and Joseph, sisters-in-law, Joan and Kelly, nephews, Brian, Mike, Kevin, and Danny, and niece, Natalie.

A lifetime of love and gratitude goes to my parents, who never pressured me to marry. They loved each other deeply and stayed married for forty-two years, until my dad died. They also had their own individual interests, and in addition to socializing as a couple, they also socialized separately with relatives and friends. They would never ever do such a thing as exclude someone because they were single. Neither of them was single at heart, but I think they both would have appreciated this book.